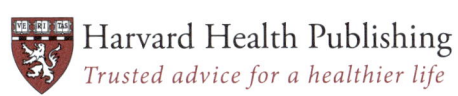 

Dear Reader,

"Hard as bone"—that's an expression we've all heard. But what does it really mean? Healthy bones are indeed hard. Your skeletal system does yeoman's work in supporting your body and facilitating your movements. But when you have osteoporosis (literally "porous bone"), you can no longer count on your skeleton to be sturdy enough to withstand even routine stress. A twist, a bend, an unexpected jolt—all can snap a dangerously weak bone. Sadly, many people have no inkling that they have been losing bone mass for years until a painful fracture of the wrist, spine, or hip brings the problem into sharp focus.

More than 10 million Americans currently live with osteoporosis, and another 43 million show early signs of bone loss. And those numbers are expected to grow as baby boomers age. According to the National Osteoporosis Foundation, an estimated 71 million Americans over age 50 are expected to have low bone density or osteoporosis by 2030, resulting in more bone fractures. The cost to the health care system will reach an estimated $25 billion per year by 2025.

For the individual, the consequences of an osteoporosis-related fracture can be devastating. Many older adults never regain the good health and quality of life they enjoyed before suffering a broken bone. Physical complications ranging from ongoing pain and stooped posture to breathing and digestive problems are common. Hip fractures can significantly impair a person's mobility, making it impossible to drive, cook, or even walk across a room without assistance.

But you don't have to wait until the damage is done to fight this disease. You can start making lifestyle changes at any age that will promote good bone health and prevent or delay severe bone loss. Ways of doing that are detailed in this report. And if you already have the disease, there have never been more options for treating it. Doctors have sophisticated tools to detect bone thinning in the earliest stages and identify people who should begin treatment and when. For those in greatest danger of an osteoporosis-related fracture, a number of highly effective medications to curb bone loss are already available, and more are on the way.

By learning about osteoporosis, you're taking a step toward better bone health. This report can help you become aware of your risk and serve as a guide for making the lifestyle changes known to reap long-term bone benefits. Regardless of your age, it's never too late—or too early—to begin boning up on bone health.

Sincerely,

David M. Slovik, M.D.
Medical Editor

Harvard Health Publishing | Harvard Medical School | 4 Blackfan Circle, 4th Floor | Boston, MA 02115

The basics of bone

Your bones are surprisingly strong. Ounce for ounce, they bear as much weight as reinforced concrete. But unlike concrete, bone isn't inert. It is a living tissue that can grow stronger in response to stresses and heal itself if injured.

Bones serve many roles in the body. They support your weight. They join forces with muscles, ligaments, and tendons to allow complex, highly articulated movements. Less obviously, they also serve as a repository of minerals that are used by the body. Like a savings bank, they allow both withdrawals and deposits of their mineral assets—a process that requires breaking down and rebuilding part of the bone matrix in order to release or absorb the minerals. Thus, even though bones seem solid and unchanging, they are in a constant state of flux, like other tissues in the body.

As you age, that process of flux inevitably includes losing some of your youthful bone mineral density (or simply, bone density—a measure of how strong your bones are). Yet osteoporosis is not inevitable. You can lose a certain amount of bone density and still be in the normal range. At a certain point, however, if the losses continue, you will be at an intermediate stage of bone loss called osteopenia, or simply low bone density. If you do not manage to halt or slow the loss at this point, you may eventually cross the line into osteoporosis, in which porous bones become weaker and more susceptible to fractures.

This report will examine both osteopenia and osteoporosis and explain the various measures you can take to help your bones, no matter which stage you are at. But first, to understand how and why osteoporosis occurs and what can be done to prevent and treat this potentially devastating ailment, it helps to know some basics about the living tissue that makes up the more than 200 individual bones of the body.

Figure 1: Compact and trabecular bone

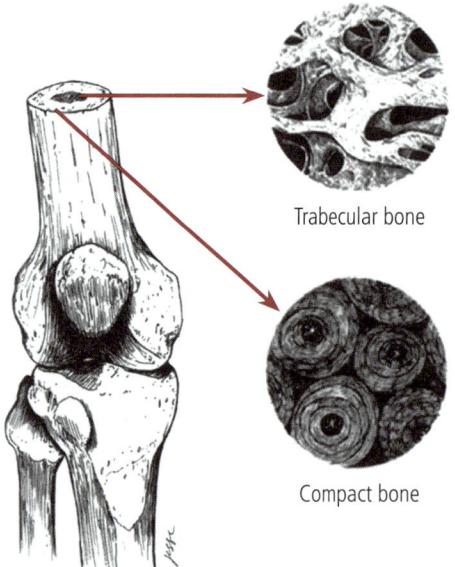

Trabecular bone

Compact bone

The bones in your body are composed of two types of tissue: compact bone and trabecular bone. Often, the compact bone—tightly packed tubes of bone tissue whose cross-sections resemble the rings of a tree trunk—forms the outer casing, while the trabecular bone, which is more porous, is found at the center.

Two types of bone tissue

The bones in your body contain two essential types of bone tissue.

Compact bone. As the name implies, compact bone tissue is densely packed. It is composed of units called osteons, which consist of tight plates wound into tubular forms that resemble rolled-up magazines (see Figure 1, at left). A tiny blood vessel, or capillary, runs through the center of each osteon, supplying nutrients and oxygen. Osteons are arranged in stacks to form a bone's hard outer casing. In fact, compact bone is sometimes referred to as cortical bone, derived from the Latin word "cortex," meaning "bark" or "shell."

Trabecular bone. The second major type of material in your skeleton is called trabecular bone, meaning "like a little beam." Trabecular bone is composed of millions of tiny beams and plates that form a lattice-like matrix (see Figure 1, page 2). It is less dense and spongier in consistency than compact bone and, for this reason, is sometimes known as spongy bone or cancellous bone (meaning "lattice-like").

Bones contain a combination of compact and trabecular tissue, with compact bone forming the dense outer casing and trabecular bone filling the interior. Over all, the ratio of compact to trabecular bone in adults is about four to one, although the proportion varies greatly from bone to bone. Long, regular bones, like those of the arms, legs, and ribs, consist primarily of compact bone. Irregularly shaped bones—such as the spinal vertebrae, pelvis, and the ends of the arm and leg bones—consist mostly of trabecular bone.

Why is this relevant? It helps explain, for example, why the spine is particularly vulnerable to osteoporosis. Not only is trabecular bone—the main constituent tissue in vertebrae—less dense than compact bone by its very nature, it is also metabolically more active, so when bones begin to lose density, trabecular bone weakens faster and therefore starts earlier in the progression toward osteoporosis. It is for this reason that trabecular bone in the spine is lost first, and why it's important to see your doctor for a bone density test of the spine no later than age 65 in women and age 70 in men, or sooner if you have risk factors.

Bone remodeling

Although compact and trabecular bone differ in structure, they are composed of the same basic material: a meshwork of protein fibers, called collagen. The collagen matrix is inlaid with calcium and phosphate minerals, which are mixed with water to form a hard, cement-like substance called hydroxyapatite. Smaller amounts of sodium, magnesium, and potassium are also present in the matrix.

Calcium, however, is the main ingredient of bone. The dynamic process by which bones take in or release this vital mineral is known as remodeling, or bone metabolism. Osteoporosis is the eventual result when bone remodeling gets out of balance, causing more calcium to leave the bones than is added.

Calcium carries a lot of weight in the body, both literally and figuratively. It's the major component of hydroxyapatite, the cement-like mineral that lends bones their strength. But it also plays a crucial role in other parts of the body. Buoyed along in the blood, calcium bustles in and out of cells, transmitting signals to nerves and muscles. In this capacity, it is vital for maintaining heart rate and blood pressure, as well as regulating internal organs.

Calcium is so important that when blood levels of this mineral drop below a certain threshold, the body raids the bones to compensate. However, the amount of calcium required to maintain all these other functions is slight—only about 1% of your body's total calcium stores. The rest—weighing about 2.25 to 4.5 pounds—is sequestered in your bones.

Tapping and replenishing calcium stores

The process by which the body removes calcium from bone is known as resorption, and it is performed by special cells called osteoclasts. The sawtooth membranes of these cells enable them to attach to the surface of bone. Once attached, they use acids and enzymes to break down the bone's matrix of collagen and minerals, releasing these materials into the bloodstream for reuse in other parts of the body. This recycling effort leaves tiny trenches in the bone (see Figure 2, page 4).

A bone-building process known as formation—carried out by cells called osteoblasts—counterbalances resorption. Osteoblasts move into the trenches left by the osteoclasts and release strands of collagen into the void. Eventually, they become trapped in the web they have woven. Held by these moorings, they evolve into structural bone cells, or osteocytes. Calcium, phosphate, and other minerals carried in the bloodstream also accumulate in the web woven by osteoblasts. The minerals coalesce into crystalline hydroxyapatite, and the formation process is complete: the bone that was removed has been fully replaced.

To maintain bone density, the body needs to keep a constant balance between bone production and breakdown. Enter the osteocytes—mature osteoblasts that have become trapped within the bone matrix they

Figure 2: The cycle of bone construction and demolition

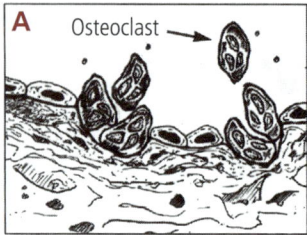
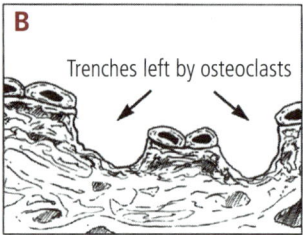
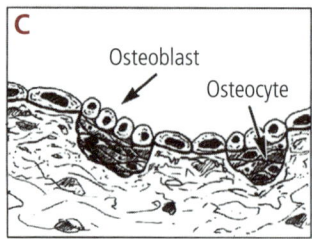
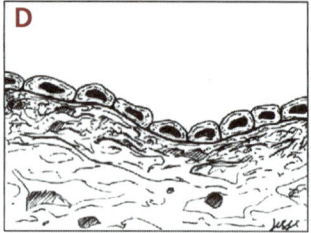

A Bone is constantly being constructed and demolished. During resorption (**A**), cells known as osteoclasts break down bone, releasing calcium into the bloodstream.

B The trenches that are left behind (**B**) are then filled in by construction cells known as osteoblasts.

C The osteoblasts release collagen into these troughs and eventually evolve into structural bone cells, or osteocytes (**C**).

D Once these osteocytes mix together with calcium, phosphate, and other minerals to form a cement-like substance known as hydroxyapatite, the process of replacing the lost bone is complete (**D**).

helped construct. Osteocytes send out signals that oversee bone remodeling. They direct osteoclasts to break down bone and osteoblasts to form new bone, thereby maintaining a kind of balance or equilibrium within the bones.

Other key players

The remodeling process releases stored calcium for vital functions elsewhere in the body, and it also keeps your skeleton fresh and healthy by replacing old bone with new. This important task in the body's housekeeping scheme requires more than just osteoclasts, osteoblasts, and osteocytes. It also takes a sizable array of hormones and other substances to carry out bone formation. For example, vitamin D (which is actually a hormone) plays a pivotal role, limiting withdrawals of calcium from bone by enhancing calcium absorption from food in the intestines into the bloodstream.

Another key player in bone health is parathyroid hormone, which is secreted by small glands behind the thyroid. The glands release parathyroid hormone when the level of calcium in the blood falls below the amount needed by the body's cells. In response, the digestive system absorbs more calcium from food and the kidneys excrete less calcium in urine, both of which help to raise blood levels of calcium. Parathyroid hormone also stimulates the osteoclasts to break down bone, releasing calcium into the bloodstream. When the blood levels are adequate, the production of parathyroid hormone falls.

The life cycle of bone

Bone remodeling is a lifelong process. At first, building outpaces demolition (resorption). Later in life the ratio is reversed. In the middle—earlier than most people realize—you reach peak bone mass, the maximum bone density you will achieve.

The early years

During the first 20 years of life, the body builds new bone more quickly than it removes old bone. By the late teens, most bone formation has already occurred. In fact, by age 20, most women have built 98% of their skeletal mass. Over the next decade, building slows, but still outpaces resorption. By age 30, most men and women reach their peak bone mass (see Figure 3, page 5). In an ideal world, you will have built strong bones early in life. But even if you haven't, it's never too late to adopt bone-preserving habits.

The density of bones at their peak varies from person to person. Heredity, lifestyle, and medical conditions all influence how much bone you'll have in the bank when heavy withdrawals begin. Following are some of the factors that influence peak bone mass.

Sex, race, and genes. In general, bone density is 30% higher in men than in women and 10% higher in blacks than in whites. Even so, there is wide variation within these groups. The difference may trace back to several genes that influence bone mass, bone turnover, and bone loss.

Diet. Nutrition early in life strongly influences bone health in adulthood. Research indicates that women whose diets contain the greatest amounts of calcium and vitamin D during childhood and adolescence have denser and stronger bones during adulthood. Consuming enough calories is also vital: when girls and women have too little body fat to support menstruation because of anorexia or bulimia, their bones suffer and they are in greater jeopardy of developing osteoporosis.

Exercise. Regular exercise contributes to peak bone density. Particularly important are weight lifting and other forms of resistance training, as well as a larger group of weight-bearing activities—that is, those in which you support your body's weight against gravity—such as running, walking, aerobics, soccer, basketball, gymnastics, tennis, and golf. Exercise puts stress on bone, and bones respond by bulking up. However, for women, exercising to an extreme can result in declining estrogen levels, amenorrhea (abnormal absence of menstrual periods), and eventually bone loss. This unhealthy situation is particularly common among young dancers, elite athletes, long-distance runners, and gymnasts.

Medications. Use of certain drugs may be accompanied by bone loss (see "Medical conditions and medications that can lead to bone loss," page 7). Too much synthetic thyroid hormone taken for an underactive thyroid gland can weaken bones. Other drugs that diminish bone strength include glucocorticoids, which are taken to control conditions such as asthma and immune disorders (see "6 ways glucocorticoids hinder bone formation," page 8), as well as medications used to treat breast and prostate cancers. Also, because several drugs that speed bone loss are commonly taken after organ transplants, people who have had these operations are at considerable risk of developing osteoporosis.

Middle age and beyond

Among women, bone mass usually remains steady until menopause, when bone is lost rapidly. But for some women, bone loss begins in the years just preceding menopause (perimenopause), as estrogen levels start to dip. While the pace of bone loss slows after the first few years of menopause, women continue to lose bone in the following years. In fact, during the five to seven years after menopause, women can lose up to 20% of their bone density.

Because androgen levels in men fall off more gradually, bone loss usually begins later for them—typically in their late 50s—and progresses more slowly. The main contributors to their bone loss are medical conditions and the general effects of aging. Men also start off with greater bone mass than women.

By ages 65 to 70, men and women lose bone at the same rate, although more women than men are diagnosed with osteoporosis at all ages. And the process can be hastened by a variety of medical conditions and medications that are covered in the next chapter.

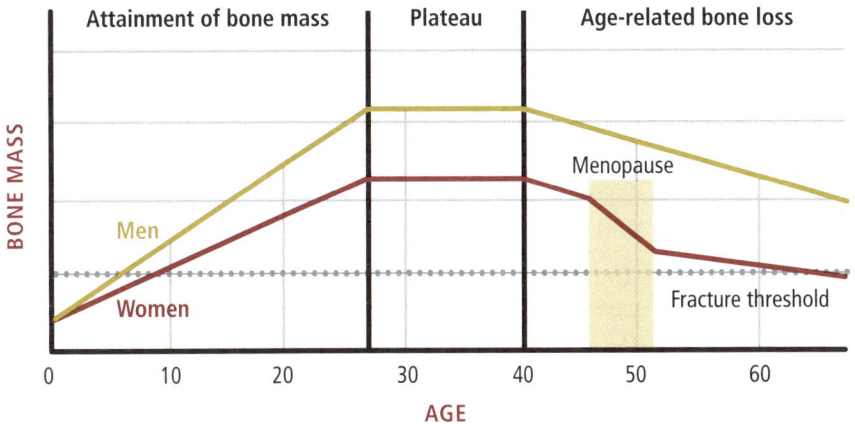

Figure 3: How bone density changes with age

Bone formation outpaces resorption up to age 30, when both men and women reach their peak bone mass. Then the process reverses, leading to a plateau and finally a loss of bone mass that occurs gradually in men but much faster in menopausal women.

Source: Clinical Endocrinology, Nov. 1990, 653–82.

What causes osteoporosis?

While a certain amount of bone loss is normal, not everyone develops osteoporosis. Many things can cause osteoporosis. Some are factors you can change. Others are beyond your control.

Bone loss begins when the cells that form bone (osteoblasts) cannot keep pace with the cells that break down bone (osteoclasts). If you were to view a microscopic video of the process, you would see the osteoclasts going about business as usual, while the osteoblasts' efforts fall short. Although the trenches dug by the osteoclasts don't get any deeper, neither are they refilled completely. As poorly filled trenches accumulate, the bone becomes thinner, more porous, and weaker than it once was, leading to a condition called osteopenia that precedes osteoporosis.

There are no symptoms associated with such bone loss. But if it continues long enough, leading to osteoporosis, bones will eventually become too weak to bear the load they were designed to carry. The result is usually a fracture of the wrist, hip, or spine.

Doctors sometimes classify osteoporosis as primary or secondary, depending on the cause.

Primary osteoporosis

The term primary osteoporosis is used to describe the most common form of the disease, which is the consequence of a normal physiological process, such as menopause or aging.

Menopause

Postmenopausal osteoporosis occurs when declining estrogen levels in women lead to rapid bone loss. Typically, the process accelerates in the first few years of menopause and then begins to level off. The effects are most prominent in trabecular bone, which isn't as dense as compact bone.

Several factors may contribute to this process. A number of researchers are examining the roles of chemical regulators, such as interleukin-1, interleukin-6, prostaglandin E2, and tumor necrosis factor, which appear to speed up bone resorption by spurring on osteoclasts as estrogen levels decline. Such research could someday lead to better drugs to prevent postmenopausal bone loss.

Aging

Gradual bone loss with aging may also lead to osteoporosis. In this case, the bone loss develops more slowly than postmenopausal osteoporosis and is usually not apparent until age 75 or later. As with all age-related changes, it probably reflects several factors.

Slowdown in bone formation. As described earlier, bone in older people is broken down more quickly than it is formed.

Reduced levels of calcium in the bloodstream. With age, the intestines gradually absorb less calcium from food, and the kidneys seem to be less efficient at conserving calcium. Thus, less calcium reaches the bloodstream, and more calcium leaves the body in feces and urine, making it increasingly likely that the body will need to tap the calcium stored in bones. To make matters worse, most people consume less calcium in their diets as they age, further straining their calcium reserves. Some older adults may avoid dairy products if they have lactose intolerance (a reduced ability to digest milk sugar), which can produce gas and abdominal discomfort. Others may shun calcium-containing foods and supplements because of their constipating effects.

Reduced vitamin D production. The body's production of vitamin D frequently drops with age as well. Your skin cells use sunlight to produce the chemical raw material that the body needs to make vitamin D. The liver and kidneys then convert this precursor into active vitamin D. However, people often spend less time in the sunlight as they grow older, so there is less of the raw material available—and in addition, the body becomes less efficient at turning this precursor into active vitamin D. Compounding the problem, many older adults consume fewer dairy products, which are fortified with vitamin D, so they take in less through their diets. Vitamin D plays a central role in the body's absorption of calcium and in the process of turning calcium into bone. If you don't have enough vitamin D to signal your intestines to absorb calcium, your body will break down bone to get the calcium it needs—no matter how much calcium you're getting from food or supplements.

Secondary osteoporosis

The term secondary osteoporosis is used to describe osteoporosis resulting from a medical condition or the use of certain medications. If you have one of these conditions or if you're taking any of these drugs, talk to your doctor about what you can do to keep your bones healthy.

Medical conditions that cause bone loss

Certain medical problems can affect bone health—some severely. For example, congenital disorders that affect bone mass over a lifetime—such as Marfan's syndrome, Ehlers-Danlos syndrome, or osteogenesis imperfecta—increase the risk for osteoporosis. Some chronic conditions, including anorexia, certain cancers, liver disease, and disorders that affect mineral absorption, may also have an impact (see "Medical conditions and medications that can lead to bone loss," below).

Medical conditions and medications that can lead to bone loss

MEDICAL CONDITIONS

- Acromegaly
- Alcoholism
- Amyloidosis
- Androgen insensitivity
- Ankylosing spondylitis
- Anorexia
- Athletic amenorrhea
- Bulimia
- Calcium deficiency
- Celiac disease
- Chronic metabolic acidosis
- Cushing's syndrome
- Cystic fibrosis
- Depression
- Diabetes (types 1 and 2)
- Ehlers-Danlos syndrome
- Emphysema
- End-stage renal disease
- Epilepsy
- Gastric bypass
- Gastrointestinal surgery
- Gaucher's disease
- Glycogen storage diseases
- Heart failure
- Hemochromatosis
- Hemophilia
- Homocystinuria
- Hypercalciuria
- Hyperprolactinemia
- Hyperthyroidism
- Hypogonadism
- Hypophosphatasia
- idiopathic scoliosis
- Inflammatory bowel disease
- Klinefelter's syndrome
- Leukemia and lymphoma
- Liver disease
- Lupus
- Malabsorptive disorders
- Marfan's syndrome
- Multiple myeloma
- Multiple sclerosis
- Muscular dystrophy
- Osteogenesis imperfecta
- Pancreatic disease
- Panhypopituitarism
- Porphyria
- Post-transplant bone disease
- Premature ovarian failure
- Primary biliary cirrhosis
- Primary hyperparathyroidism
- Renal tubular acidosis
- Rheumatoid arthritis
- Sarcoidosis
- Sickle cell disease
- Systemic mastocytosis
- Thalassemia
- Thyrotoxicosis
- Turner's syndrome

MEDICATIONS WITH DEFINITE LINKS TO BONE LOSS

- Anti-androgens
- Aromatase inhibitors
- Glucocorticoids

MEDICATIONS WITH POSSIBLE LINKS TO BONE LOSS

- Anticonvulsants
- Barbiturates
- Canagliflozin (Invokana)
- Cyclosporine (Neoral, Sandimmune, others)
- Depot medroxyprogesterone (Depo-Provera)
- Gonadotropin-releasing hormone agonists
- Heparin (long-term therapy)
- Lithium
- Loop diuretics
- Methotrexate
- Proton-pump inhibitors (PPIs)
- Selective serotonin reuptake inhibitors (SSRIs)
- Tacrolimus (Hecoria, Prograf, others)
- Thiazolidinediones (TZDs)
- Thyroid hormone (in excessive doses)

So does primary hyperparathyroidism, a condition in which people have abnormally high levels of parathyroid hormone. This hormone helps regulate the amount of calcium in the blood. Excessive levels spur the removal of calcium from bones and increase the amount of calcium in the blood. In turn, the kidneys often try to compensate for the extraordinarily high blood levels of calcium by excreting large amounts of it in the urine. Every year, approximately 100,000 new cases are detected, most of them in women. Often, this condition has no symptoms and is found only when a routine blood test shows high calcium levels. However, as primary hyperparathyroidism advances, it can cause kidney stones, muscle weakness, fatigue, and eventually osteoporosis.

Medications that cause bone loss

A variety of medications, both prescription drugs and those available over the counter, can affect bone strength and possibly raise the risk of suffering a harmful fracture. In an otherwise healthy person, such medications might have a small effect that doesn't unduly raise fracture risk. But if you have already begun to lose bone or you've been diagnosed with osteoporosis, the effects of these drugs may be enough of a concern to warrant discussing them with your doctor. You and your doctor can decide whether you should stay on these drugs or switch off them based on your bone health and overall health.

Researchers have found a definitive link between the following drugs and bone loss:

Glucocorticoids. The most common cause of drug-related osteoporosis is the use of glucocorticoids, also known as corticosteroids (see "6 ways glucocorticoids hinder bone formation," above right). These drugs, which include prednisone, are often used to treat conditions such as asthma, rheumatoid arthritis, and chronic obstructive pulmonary disease. Glucocorticoids are also used to prevent rejection after organ transplantation. Although inhaled corticosteroids, which are an integral part of asthma treatment, are less likely to cause bone loss than oral corticosteroids, they can still weaken bones, especially at high doses.

Aromatase inhibitors (for women). Many women with breast cancer have benefited from a class of drugs called aromatase inhibitors, which block estrogen production. These drugs include anastrozole (Arimidex), exemestane (Aromasin), and letrozole (Femara). These drugs reduce the chance of cancer coming back in women whose cancers are estrogen-positive, meaning they tend to grow in response to estrogen. Aromatase inhibitors are more effective than tamoxifen (Nolvadex, Apo-Tamox, Tamofen, Tamone), a leading cancer drug, in preventing cancer recurrence after treatment. But because estrogen slows bone loss, lowering levels of this hormone with an aromatase inhibitor can harm bone health. As a result, women taking these drugs are at greater risk of spinal and other fractures.

Androgen-suppressing drugs (for men). Certain men with prostate cancer undergo androgen deprivation therapy with a variety of different medications that lower levels of male hormones to suppress the cancer. But at the same time, androgen deprivation therapy can put them at greater risk of bone loss and fractures. In one study, about 20% of men undergoing this therapy who survived for at least five years experienced a bone fracture, compared with 13% of men who did not receive this treatment.

Medications that might cause bone loss

There is a lengthy list of drugs with possible links to bone loss (see "Medical conditions and medications that can lead to bone loss," page 7). The following are some with a stronger linkage, although the effect has not been proved yet.

▶ 6 ways glucocorticoids hinder bone formation

These medications—including prednisone, methylprednisolone, and hydrocortisone—do the following:

1. Interfere with the body's ability to absorb calcium from food
2. Increase the amount of calcium lost in the urine
3. Fuel bone-destroying osteoclasts
4. Hamper bone-building osteoblasts
5. Possibly trigger the body to produce too much parathyroid hormone, which removes calcium from bone stores
6. Reduce the production of estrogen in women and testosterone in men.

Anticonvulsants. Numerous studies have found an increased risk of bone loss and fractures among people who take drugs called anticonvulsants, which are used primarily to prevent epileptic seizures. The strongest risks have been linked with older anticonvulsant drugs known as enzyme inducers: carbamazepine (Tegretol), phenobarbital (Luminal), phenytoin (Dilantin), and primidone (Mysoline). Valproate (Depakote), another older drug, also has been linked with higher risk. There's less research on newer anticonvulsants, including gabapentin (Neurontin), lamotrigine (Lamictal), levetiracetam (Keppra), topiramate (Topamax), and vigabatrin (Sabril). The Epilepsy Foundation recommends paying close attention to general guidelines for prevention of osteoporosis, including regular weight-bearing exercise and sufficient intake of vitamin D and calcium.

Diabetes drugs. Doctors have noticed bone fractures—as well as reductions in the bone density of the hip and lower spine—in people taking the diabetes drug canagliflozin (Invokana), which is used to lower blood sugar in people with type 2 diabetes. In the fall of 2015, the FDA added a warning about bone loss to the label of canagliflozin. (Canagliflozin belongs to a class of drugs called SGLT2 inhibitors. But so far, the FDA warning applies only to canagliflozin.) The fractures that prompted the warning occurred as soon as 12 weeks after beginning the drug. Another class of diabetes drugs called thiazolidinediones (TZDs), which includes pioglitazone (Actos) and rosiglitazone (Avandia), has also been linked to increased bone loss and fracture risk. Before you start taking one of these drugs, it may be worth discussing the bone risks with your doctor.

Proton-pump inhibitors (PPIs). This popular class of medications, used to reduce stomach acid, may erode bone strength and increase the risk of fractures. (Omeprazole, marketed as Prilosec, is one of the best-known PPIs.) By reducing stomach acid, PPIs may also impair the absorption of calcium from food, potentially leading to weaker bones and a greater risk of bone fractures. Research to date suggests that the effect, if it is real, is modest, though not all studies agree. However, in a person already at risk of low bone density or fractures, long-term use of PPIs could pose a legitimate concern.

If you're at risk for fractures and you use a PPI for heartburn or to prevent ulcer flare-ups, ask your doctor how to counterbalance the effect of the PPI. If you take calcium supplements, you may want to switch to a product with calcium citrate, which does not require stomach acid for absorption (unlike calcium carbonate, which does require acid for maximal absorption). Calcium citrate is often recommended for people taking PPIs long-term.

Antidepressants. Researchers have uncovered a possible association between reduced bone strength and a class of antidepressants called selective serotonin reuptake inhibitors (SSRIs). These drugs may contribute to bone loss by enhancing the effects of osteoclasts. However, the link is far from certain. Although people who use SSRIs seem to have a modestly higher risk of fractures, it's not possible yet to show a definite cause-and-effect connection. In the meantime, if you are taking these medications long-term at your doctor's recommendation, you may want to discuss whether there is more you could do to protect yourself against fractures, such as being screened for low bone density or increasing your calcium, vitamin D, and exercise.

Organ transplant drugs. Some medications, such as cyclosporine (Neoral, Sandimmune) and tacrolimus (Hecoria, Prograf), that are used to prevent organ rejection after transplants may also further bone loss. People using any of these medications should be vigilant about protecting their bones. They should pay special attention to diet and exercise and consider other steps—such as taking osteoporosis drugs (see "Protecting your bones: Medication," page 38)—to prevent bone loss and fractures.

Diuretics. Diuretics, or "water pills," make the body excrete water and salt. They are often used to treat high blood pressure. Those in the group known as loop diuretics cause the kidneys to release more calcium. Commonly prescribed loop diuretics that have this effect include ethacrynic acid (Edecrin) and furosemide (Lasix). Several studies have shown that people who take loop diuretics have slightly lower bone density in fracture danger zones like the hip, and a greater overall fracture risk.

Know your risk factors

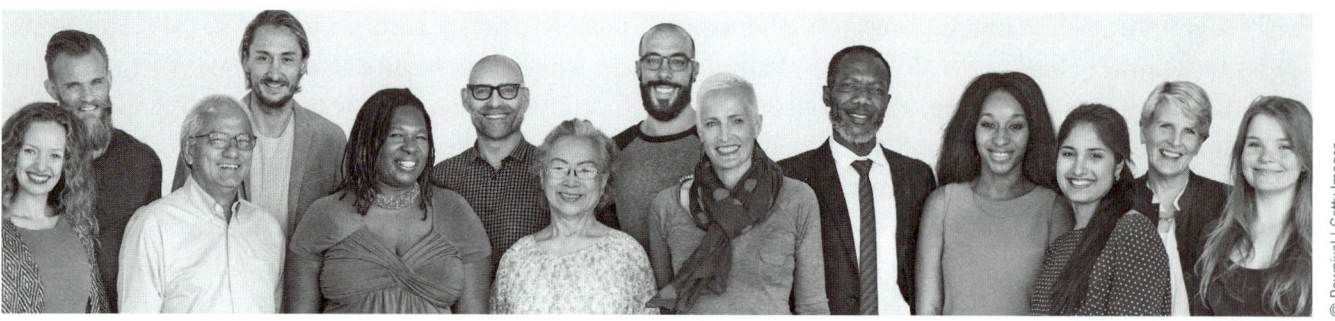

Women generally face a higher risk for osteoporosis than men, but two million men have the disease and 12 million more are at risk for it.

Certain factors make you more vulnerable to developing the bone weakening that can lead to fractures (see Figure 4, page 11). Some of these risk factors—like age and family history—aren't within your control. Others are modifiable with some relatively simple lifestyle changes.

If you haven't yet been diagnosed with osteoporosis, use these risk factors as a guide to launching a discussion about bone density testing with your doctor. If you have already been diagnosed, addressing the lifestyle factors you can change can help preserve the bone strength you still have.

Risk factors you can't control

Though you can't change these factors, awareness of your risks can motivate you to start protecting your bones before they are dangerously weakened.

Gender. For a variety of reasons, women are at higher risk than men, though men can develop osteoporosis, too (see "Osteoporosis risk in women," page 11, and "Osteoporosis risk in men," page 12).

Aging. Advancing years inevitably bring a higher risk for osteoporosis—particularly for women. According to the CDC, 16% of women and 4% of men ages 50 and over have osteoporosis as measured at the neck of the femur (near where the thighbone connects to the hip) or the lumbar spine (the vertebrae of the lower back). Other people in this age group typically show signs of low bone strength in the spine or femoral neck, making them more likely to eventually develop osteoporosis.

Family history of the disease. The genetic traits you inherit also strongly influence your risk. Between 70% and 80% of bone structure is genetically determined. Both men and women whose first-degree family members (parents, siblings) have had fractures are at greater risk. In fact, a woman whose mother or father had a fracture is at twice the risk of a break—regardless of her measured bone density.

Race. Caucasian and Asian women face the highest osteoporosis risk, because their bones tend to be thinner and smaller than those of African American and Hispanic women. Asian women also tend to have a lower dietary intake of calcium, because many of them are lactose intolerant. Yet surprisingly, despite having thinner bones, Asian women are less likely to fracture a hip than white women. This lower risk may be due to anatomical differences in the hip bone.

Risk factors you can control

A poor diet, lack of exercise, smoking, and alcohol use can all hasten the development of osteopenia or osteoporosis as you age. If you've already been diagnosed with bone loss, addressing these risks can help protect and preserve the integrity of your bones for as long as possible.

Inadequate calcium and vitamin D levels. Inadequate intake of calcium from your diet—as well as conditions that may interfere with calcium absorption by the intestines—leads to lower calcium levels in the blood. The body compensates by releasing calcium from the bones, which weakens them. Your body needs vitamin D to properly absorb calcium, so adequate amounts of this vitamin are also necessary.

Sedentary lifestyle. When you are at rest, bone formation slows; when you are physically active, bones bulk up and become stronger. The research to date suggests that leading a physically active life can decrease the risk of having a fracture in the spine or hip by 30% to 50%.

Smoking. Smokers tend to lose bone faster than nonsmokers. Smoking may both interfere with the absorption of calcium and lower the amount of bone-protective estrogen the body produces. A number of studies, some of them quite large, have found that men and women who smoked were at greater risk of breaking a hip or other bone. In fact, a report from the U.S. Surgeon General on osteoporosis noted that smokers are 55% more likely than nonsmokers to break a hip.

Excess alcohol consumption. The amount of alcohol you drink can affect your bone health. Alcohol may interfere with the body's ability to convert inactive vitamin D into its active form. It also appears to hamper bone formation and increase losses of calcium and magnesium from the body. Excessive drinking may be accompanied by poor nutrition and an increased tendency to fall. People who consume more than two drinks per day may be at moderately higher risk of low bone density and fractures, compared with nondrinkers.

Medications. As described earlier in this report (see "Secondary osteoporosis," page 7), some drugs contribute to bone loss, raising the risk for osteoporosis. If you're taking a medication known to affect bone density, talk to your doctor about what steps you may need to take to keep your bones healthy.

Osteoporosis risk in women

Women are more likely than men to develop osteoporosis because they have smaller skeletons, their bone loss begins earlier and occurs more rapidly, and they have a lower peak bone density to begin with. About 80% of the 10 million Americans with osteoporosis are women. The Study of Osteoporotic Fractures—a landmark National Institutes of Health study of almost 10,000 women ages 65 and older—found that, on average, bone mass fell by approximately 5% every five years in women after age 65.

The study looked at characteristics that are significantly more common among women who have osteoporosis. Together with other research, it provides a good idea of some factors that predispose certain women to the condition, in addition to the general risk factors above:

- Small-boned, thin women tend to have lower bone density and a higher risk of fractures. It may be because their bones are smaller, but science doesn't give us a definite answer on this point. In the Study of Osteoporotic Fractures, women 65 and older with the smallest body size had twice the rate of hip fractures (10 in 1,000) compared with the rate among the largest women in the study (five in 1,000).
- Because estrogen slows bone resorption, women who are past menopause and those who have had their ovaries removed are at higher risk. So are younger women who have too little body fat (sometimes because of excessive exercise, anorexia, or

Figure 4: A fragile state

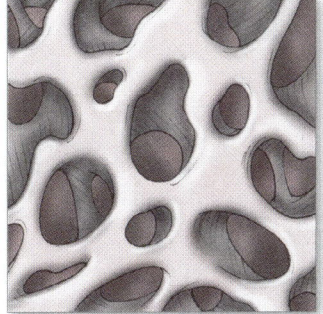
Normal, healthy bone

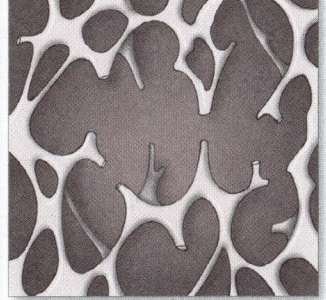
Osteoporotic bone

Osteoporotic bone is more porous and less dense than healthy bone. The result is bone that is more fragile and more vulnerable to breaks. Areas that are particularly vulnerable include the vertebrae and the femoral head (the top of the thighbone).

bulimia) and consequently too little estrogen to menstruate regularly.

Talk to your doctor about your risk and what, if anything, you should do about it, including having a bone density evaluation. The National Osteoporosis Foundation recommends routine dual energy x-ray absorptiometry (DEXA or DXA) testing for women starting at age 65 to measure bone density. (For a more complete list of screening guidelines, see "Who should be screened?" on page 17.)

Osteoporosis risk in men

It is a persistent misperception that osteoporosis is a "women's disease." Although bone loss strikes women younger and harder, men, too, are at significant risk of low bone density and the harmful fractures that can follow (see Figure 5, below). According to the National Osteoporosis Foundation, two million American men have osteoporosis and about 12 million more are at risk. Each year, about 80,000 men break a hip—and when they do, they are two to three times more likely to die of complications from their injuries than women are.

Nonetheless, men constitute only 20% of Americans with osteoporosis. Two factors make men less vulnerable than women to bone loss: they have greater bone density at skeletal maturity, and they experience a more gradual decline in hormone levels. When men under age 75 develop osteoporosis, it's often because of an underlying health condition. In these cases, treatments address the condition or conditions that are responsible.

But "less vulnerable" does not mean "invulnerable," and the reason comes right back to declining sex hormones. Experts believe that age-related declines in testosterone levels may cause bone loss. Men also produce estrogen (though in smaller quantities than women), and declining estrogen with aging may be as significant a factor as low testosterone. In the Osteoporotic Fractures in Men Study, which involved over 2,400 men 65 and older, men who had low levels of both testosterone and estrogen were more likely to have osteoporosis than those with normal levels of these hormones. Researchers have also found that men with low hormone levels are more likely to fracture a hip.

The National Osteoporosis Foundation recommends routine DEXA testing for men starting at age 70 to measure bone density. Men ages 50 to 69 should also be tested if they have risk factors for osteoporosis, such as a history of a previous fracture, low body weight, or smoking. The Endocrine Society has issued a clinical practice guideline that recommends the same level of osteoporosis screening for men as for women. However, the U.S. Preventive Services Task Force, an independent panel of experts, concluded that "the current evidence is insufficient to assess the balance of benefits and harms of screening for osteoporosis in men."

There is one thing that all experts agree on, however: men should protect their bones by following the same lifestyle recommendations suggested for women. That means engaging in regular weight-bearing and strengthening exercises, getting adequate amounts of calcium and vitamin D from food and (if needed) supplements, and avoiding habits known to deplete bone mass, such as smoking and drinking excessive amounts of alcohol. These habits will help maintain a solid reserve of bone mass to ward off fractures later in life.

Figure 5: Fracture risk

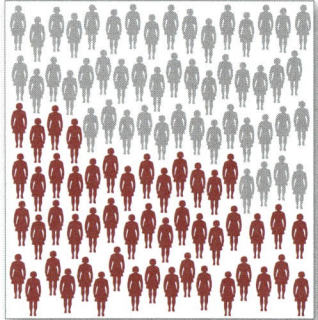
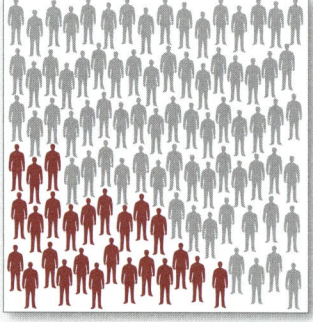

▲ **FOR WOMEN**
50% risk: One out of two women over age 50 will have an osteoporosis-related fracture in her lifetime.

▲ **FOR MEN**
25% risk: One out of four men over age 50 will have an osteoporosis-related fracture in his lifetime.

The consequences of osteoporosis

Osteoporosis was once known as a silent disease because it gives no warning signs as it gnaws away at bones. Eventually, it would make itself known when a break occurred without due cause, perhaps triggered by something as innocent as a sneeze.

Although any bone can be affected, most breaks related to osteoporosis occur in one of three sites: the hip, the spine, or the wrist. Fractures at these sites, particularly in women who are past menopause, are most common because these regions contain relatively high proportions of trabecular bone and are therefore especially vulnerable to the effects of bone loss.

Osteoporotic fractures exact a high toll, leaving some people in pain while stripping others of their ability to perform everyday activities or to move around independently. Three in five people who break a hip because of osteoporosis will never fully regain their previous level of functioning. Many people become so fearful of breaking another bone that they limit their activities, which causes them to feel helpless, isolated, and depressed. Research has shown that fractures in the spine, hip, and thighbone have the greatest impact on quality of life.

Hip fractures

About one in seven osteoporosis-related fractures occurs at the hip. Typically, these are the most serious osteoporotic fractures. Hip fractures usually involve the neck or the intertrochanteric region of the thighbone (see Figure 6, at right). Breaks can also occur in bones of the pelvis. The impact of a hip fracture on someone's life and activity level depends in large part on the person's physical condition and other medical issues.

At best, the breaks are temporarily immobilizing, requiring confinement to bed or a wheelchair. Surgery is usually needed but may not be feasible because of other disorders, such as heart or lung disease, which increase the risk for complications following an operation. As a result, the damaged bone often heals badly, resulting in permanent disability.

The injury often has devastating effects on mobility and independence. Six out of 10 people who break a hip never fully regain their former level of independence. Some are permanently less able to perform ordinary daily activities, such as dressing themselves or rising from a chair. Even walking across a room may be difficult. These changes in mobility and daily functioning can make it necessary to seek home health care or to move to a facility that can provide care. Half of the people who suffer a hip or spine fracture will need assistance walking, and one in four will need long-term nursing home care.

While people seldom die directly from a hip fracture, this injury and its accompanying medical problems can trigger a downward spiral in health. Complications, such as pneumonia or blood clots,

Figure 6: Common hip fractures

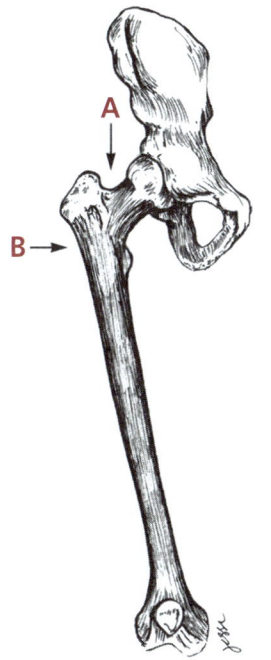

Most hip fractures occur in the top portion of the thighbone (femur)—either at the femoral neck (**A**) or at the intertrochanteric region (**B**).

Each year there are nearly 300,000 hip fractures from osteoporosis in the United States. Fracturing a hip can have serious consequences, such as impairing the ability to walk or to perform simple everyday chores, and the resulting immobility can lead to a downward spiral in health.

that result from the fracture itself or surgery to treat it are sometimes fatal. One in five people who have a hip fracture dies in the first year after the injury. The risk of death is 10% to 20% in the first six months after a fracture in the hip or spine. Fractures are particularly deadly among nursing home residents and people with cognitive impairment or other health issues. The risk of death also disproportionately affects people ages 80 and older, who are 10 to 15 times more likely to fracture a hip than people 60 to 65. Those who do survive may have trouble living on their own.

But there is some encouraging news, too. According to a 2015 study of Medicare claims, the hip fracture rate declined each year from 2002 to 2012. However, this plateaued at levels higher than expected for years 2013, 2014, and 2015 resulting in an estimated increase of more than 11,000 hip fractures during that time period. In sum, the dangers of a hip fracture remain a powerful incentive to do all you can to preserve your bone health.

Spinal (vertebral) fractures

Fractures in the spine are much more common than hip fractures. Unlike hip fractures, spinal fractures often occur without a traumatic cause like a fall. Even so, these injuries can be quite debilitating.

Simple acts of daily life, such as bending over, twisting, coughing, or lifting, can be enough to collapse a vertebra weakened by osteoporosis. In such cases, the bones of the spine, which consist primarily of trabecular bone, aren't broken in the usual sense of the term. Rather than being snapped like twigs—as in the case of a broken arm or leg—the vertebrae are compressed, in the same way that a paper cup would be flattened when stepped on. Figure 7 (at left) shows the effects of compression fractures on the spine. Vertebral fractures can cause a loss of height and, more seriously, spinal deformation—either a rounding of the back (dorsal kyphosis, sometimes called dowager's hump), a sideways curvature of the spine (scoliosis), or a combination of the two (kyphoscoliosis).

Compression fractures may be accompanied by pain that is sharp, dull, intense, or radiating around the side. Pain may also come from spasms in the muscles at the sides of the spine. It may come and go for several months, often recurring after the person sits in the same position for a long time. Discomfort from fractures can usually be relieved with pain medications such as aspirin or ibuprofen (Advil, Motrin).

In many instances, vertebral fractures cause little or no pain. The principal clue that they have occurred is a gradual shrinkage or stooped posture. The amount of height lost and the degree of deformity will depend on the number, location, and severity of the compression fractures. However, narrowing of the cushion-like discs between vertebrae—which often occurs as part of aging—may also cause deformity and a loss of height.

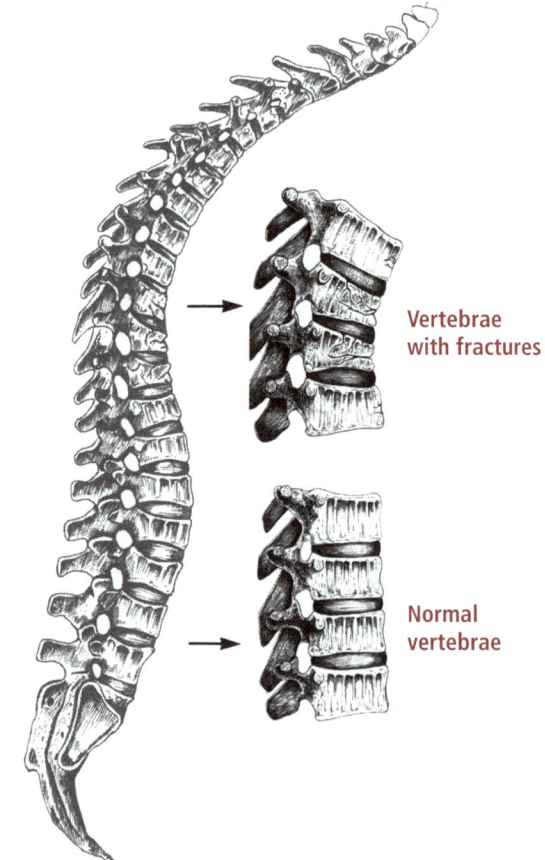

Figure 7: A look at normal and compressed vertebrae

Normal vertebrae are upright, but if several vertebrae collapse, it can cause a curvature of the spinal column known as dorsal kyphosis, or dowager's hump. This condition can make it difficult to walk without a cane or walker and can interfere with proper breathing and digestion.

Can hip protectors prevent breaks?

A quick online search will turn up plenty of hip pads that are touted as a way to help prevent a hip fracture if you fall. The pads, which consist of a stiff plastic shield underlaid with foam padding, are meant to be strapped onto the hip.

For people living in nursing homes, who are at high risk of a fracture, some studies suggest hip protectors may reduce injuries. But scientific reviews of the best research available have failed to prove that providing hip protectors to older adults living independently reduces the incidence of hip fractures.

The main challenge is getting people to wear the hip protectors consistently and properly. The pads can be uncomfortable and awkward, and many people just don't like wearing them. Also, people may fall in circumstances in which they would not be wearing the pads, for example in the bath or shower. But if worn consistently by people at risk of hip fracture, these pads could theoretically be of benefit.

Most people who have vertebral fractures have one or two, most commonly in the thoracic, or mid-back, region. While one or two mid-back compression fractures may produce only a slight loss of height, having many of them can profoundly affect your appearance, mobility, and health. As the number of fractures increases, the spine becomes progressively more distorted. The upper body is thrust down and forward. The abdominal muscles sag, and the space between the ribs and pelvis closes. The chest wall becomes cramped, and the abdominal organs are compressed and pushed forward. Breathing may become difficult and digestion may be impaired, leading to bloating and heartburn.

Severe spinal deformity affects mobility almost as significantly as a hip fracture. Since walking erect is difficult, a cane or walker becomes essential. Riding in a car for more than a few minutes can be very uncomfortable. Two procedures—vertebroplasty and kyphoplasty (see page 50)—can stabilize compressed vertebrae, relieve pain, and improve daily functioning.

Wrist fractures

Osteoporosis accounts for nearly 400,000 wrist fractures a year. These breaks are usually the result of an attempt to break a fall. Typically, the force of the impact snaps the end of the radius, the long bone that runs from the elbow to the thumb, often producing a characteristic break known as a Colles' fracture. Normally, after a wrist fracture occurs, the arm is immobilized in a cast, splint, or sling and allowed to heal, although surgery is sometimes needed. Wrist fractures usually mend completely. However, they occasionally result in deformity and a loss of some function that interferes with the ability to perform everyday activities with ease.

Other consequences

Although trabecular bone loses strength more rapidly, compact bone eventually becomes vulnerable as well. As osteoporosis advances, bones with a high proportion of compact tissue—such as the pelvis, tibia (shin), humerus (upper arm), and femur (thigh)—are fractured with increasing frequency. Ribs may be broken from the force of a cough.

Although the jawbone may not snap, it is not exempt from bone loss. As the jaw becomes increasingly porous, it provides less support for the teeth anchored into it. The result can be dental problems such as loose teeth and ill-fitting dental plates.

Detecting osteoporosis

In the past, osteoporosis was frequently diagnosed only after a bone fracture. For many people, that diagnosis came too late to be of much use. Today, osteoporosis can be detected earlier with a bone mineral density test. Such a test can also provide information regarding your risk of suffering a fracture and can help you and your doctor monitor your progress if you're taking bone-building medications.

DEXA scans for bone density

Several technologies can assess bone density, but the most common is dual energy x-ray absorptiometry (DEXA), which has been around for over 30 years. For this procedure, a machine sends x-rays through bones in order to calculate bone density. The process is quick, taking only five minutes. And it's simple: you lie on a table while a scanner passes over your body (see Figure 8, below). While this technology can measure bone density at any spot in the body, it is usually used for three readings in particular—the lumbar spine (in the lower back), total hip (a specific site near the hip joint), and femoral neck (the top of the thighbone, or femur; see Figure 6, page 13). DEXA accomplishes this with only one-tenth of the radiation exposure of a standard chest x-ray.

DEXA is considered the gold standard for osteoporosis screening. Ultrasound, which uses sound waves to measure bone density at the heel, shin, or finger, is sometimes used at health fairs and in some medical offices where DEXA may not be available. Quantitative computed tomography can also be used to measure bone density in the spine and hip.

Bone density tests will give you a number called a T-score, which represents how close you are to average peak bone density. The World Health Organization has established the following classification system:
- If your T-score is –1 or greater: your bone density is considered normal.
- If your T-score is between –1 and –2.5: you have low bone density, known as osteopenia, but not osteoporosis.
- If your T-score is –2.5 or less: you have osteoporosis, even if you haven't yet broken a bone.

Once you know your T score, you can also calculate your FRAX score, which tells you your likelihood of breaking a bone in the next 10 years (see "How likely are you to break a bone? Your FRAX score and more," page 18).

Vertebral fracture assessment

Because vertebral fractures are so common in older adults, and they often occur with no symptoms to warn of their presence, the National Osteoporosis Foundation recommends vertebral imaging at the same time as the DEXA test for certain groups of people. A vertebral fracture assessment (VFA) uses the same type of x-ray as DEXA, but instead of measuring bone density, it shows the shape of the ver-

Figure 8: Scanning for osteoporosis

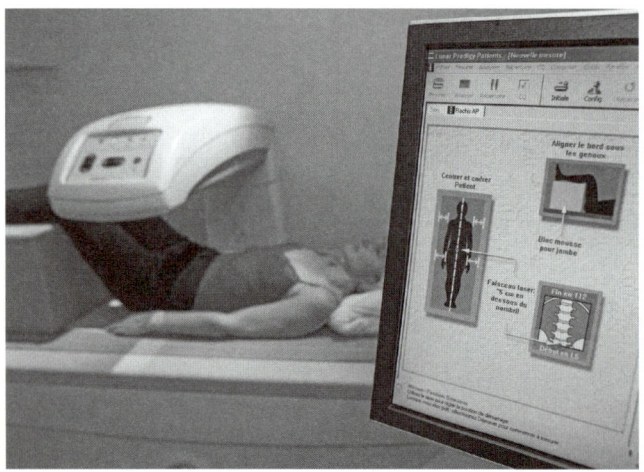

Dual energy x-ray absorptiometry (DEXA) is the most common method of detecting osteoporosis today. Most physicians consider it the most accurate diagnostic procedure.

Who should be screened?

Screenings for osteoporosis are not routinely given to everyone; instead, they are done on a case-by-case basis. Experts are still debating who should receive bone density screening, and it remains unclear whether the benefits of tests such as dual energy x-ray absorptiometry (DEXA) justify the cost of testing everyone. Talk to your doctor about whether testing is right for you.

Consider being screened if you are

- a woman age 65 or older or a man age 70 or older
- a postmenopausal woman under age 65 or a man age 50 to 70 with one or more risk factors for osteoporosis
- a woman or man with a medical condition or taking a medication that places you at high risk for osteoporotic fractures
- a woman in menopausal transition with specific risk factors for fractures (such as low body weight or a prior fracture)
- a woman or man who has fractured a bone after age 50
- a woman or man who has taken glucocorticoids for at least two months.

However, it's important to note that coverage varies among insurance plans. Some plans may refuse to pay for a DEXA scan. Others might specify how often you can have this test. For example, Medicare will cover the cost of one bone density test every two years, or more often if your doctor deems it medically necessary. So that you don't wind up footing the bill yourself, it pays to check with your plan first.

tebrae. The goal is to see if any of the vertebrae are deformed—a possible sign of fracture. More vertebrae are scanned in a VFA than in a traditional DEXA test for bone density. If the VFA shows that you have one or more fractures, you likely have severe osteoporosis and will need more aggressive treatment.

VFA is recommended for
- women ages 70 and older and men ages 80 and older with a T-score of –1 or less at the lumbar spine, total hip, or femoral neck
- women ages 65 to 69 and men ages 70 to 79 with a T-score of –1.5 or less at the lumbar spine, total hip, or femoral neck
- women and men ages 50 and older with risks such as a fracture during adulthood, total height loss of 1.5 inches or more, recent height loss of 0.8 inches or more, and recent or long-term glucocorticoid treatment.

Tests of bone quality

Although DEXA remains the tool of choice for assessing bone mineral density—the volume of minerals within bone—some newer measurements assess another aspect of bone: the quality. There's no precise definition of bone quality, but it includes the structure, or architecture, at a microscopic level and any microscopic fractures. Bone quality is important to the extent that it reflects the strength of bone and its resistance to fracture.

Researchers in recent years have developed ways of estimating bone quality. Perhaps the best known is the trabecular bone score (TBS). TBS estimates the quality of trabecular bone and how vulnerable it is to fracture. The score is calculated using an algorithm that interprets the shading in a DEXA scan, in which microscopic breaks show up as dark gray or black.

Research suggests that TBS helps predict fracture risk independently of DEXA and FRAX results. The International Society for Clinical Densitometry says TBS can be used along with these tests to adjust estimates of fracture risk for women after menopause and for men over age 50. However, this technology is relatively new and may not be covered by insurance.

Other tools are being developed to assess bone quality using noninvasive techniques.

Lab tests for bone turnover

Your doctor may use blood and urine tests to check for secondary causes of osteoporosis. In addition, these tests can provide information about bone turnover, the rate at which bone is remodeled. The tests measure substances called biochemical markers that are released during bone formation and resorption. High levels of biomarkers associated with bone resorption can indicate high bone turnover, a red flag for declining bone health.

A doctor might also order one of these tests to assess your response to treatment. For example, a

How likely are you to break a bone? Your FRAX score and more

While bone density tests can identify people who are at greater risk for fractures, they aren't the only predictors. A tool developed by the World Health Organization calculates an individual's real-life risk of suffering an osteoporosis-related fracture in the coming years. FRAX (which stands for fracture risk assessment tool) incorporates bone density scores with other weighted risk factors to arrive at a percent probability that a person will break a hip or suffer another type of osteoporotic fracture such as a break in the vertebra, forearm, or shoulder within 10 years. Risk factors used are age, sex, height, weight, previous fragility fracture as an adult, parental history of hip fracture, current smoking, alcohol use (three or more drinks per day), glucocorticoid use for more than three months, rheumatoid arthritis, and secondary osteoporosis.

The FRAX score is calculated for people whose bone density is in the range for osteopenia (T-score between –1 and –2.5). It was developed to help physicians better identify high-risk individuals in this group. If you've had a bone density test or if you think you might have an increased risk of osteoporosis, you may want to ask your physician about calculating your FRAX score. The tool is geared for doctors' use, but you can find it online at www.shef.ac.uk/FRAX. Based in part on the FRAX tool, the National Osteoporosis Foundation recommends that doctors consider drug therapy for men and women ages 50 and over who meet one or more of the following criteria:

- a previous hip or spinal fracture
- a T-score of –2.5 or less at the hip or spine
- a T-score between –1 and –2.5 at the hip or spine together with a 10-year FRAX-estimated risk of at least 20% for a major fracture or 3% for a hip fracture.

Watch for these red flags

If you don't know your bone density measurement or FRAX score, familiarize yourself with the factors that increase your chance of falling and breaking a bone. If any of the following red flags apply to you, address them and discuss them with your doctor as appropriate:

- low levels of physical activity
- overall weakness and frailty
- low muscle mass or impaired strength
- advancing age
- excessive alcohol use
- a history of falls
- balance problems
- poor eyesight
- taking medications (such as sedatives and blood pressure drugs) that can cause dizziness, lightheadedness, or impaired balance
- hazards such as electrical cords or throw rugs cluttering the walking paths around your house.

urine test revealing that bone turnover slowed after you started taking an osteoporosis drug could be a sign that the treatment is working. Conversely, if tests show that the rate of bone turnover has remained the same or increased, it may suggest that the treatment is ineffective (or that you are not taking your medication). Your doctor should find out what's going on and determine the best course of action, which may include adjusting your dose or offering suggestions to ensure that you take your medicine as prescribed.

The bottom line on lab tests for bone turnover is this: Doctors don't routinely use these tests to diagnose osteoporosis or predict fracture risk—DEXA is the best tool for that job. But they may be helpful under certain circumstances when bone turnover needs to be assessed.

Developing a plan of action

If you've been diagnosed with osteopenia or osteoporosis, your doctor will help you develop a plan to slow bone destruction and possibly even gain back a little of the bone you've lost. That plan will likely include three main strategies: diet, exercise, and medication. A fourth strategy—fall prevention—won't slow bone destruction, but like the first three strategies, it helps lessen the chances of a devastating fracture. You'll find more detail on these strategies in later chapters.

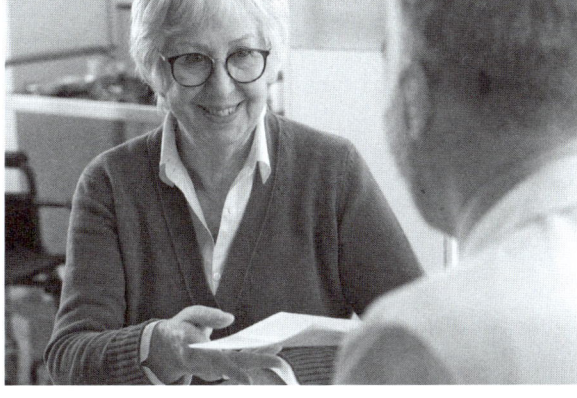

Your doctor will help you develop a plan to maintain as much bone density as possible and maybe even build a little bone strength. The main strategies are diet, exercise, and medication.

If you have osteopenia (T-score between –1 and –2.5)

According to your T-score, your bone density is lower than normal, but your fracture risk isn't as high as that of someone with osteoporosis. However, you are still at increased risk for fractures, as many fractures occur in this group. You may not need medicines at this point, and you won't necessarily progress to osteoporosis. A few lifestyle interventions should slow down the rate of bone loss and may even help you regain a small amount of bone, although they won't restore you to youthful bone density.

To protect your bones, your doctor will likely suggest the following:

Exercise. Staying active slows bone loss, strengthens the muscles that support your skeleton, and improves your coordination and balance so you're less likely to fall. A combination of strength training (weight training) and weight-bearing exercises (walking, tennis, stair climbing) is ideal for preserving bones. The stress on bones from these types of exercise causes your body to keep reinforcing the bones.

Get enough calcium and vitamin D. These nutrients are important for both fall and fracture prevention. Ask your doctor whether you can get enough calcium and vitamin D from your diet alone or if you need to take a supplement.

Quit smoking. This habit, which is also bad for your heart, lungs, skin, and other organs, can increase your fracture risk. Ask your doctor about nicotine replacement products, medicines, and other strategies to help you kick the habit.

Don't drink too much alcohol. Excess alcohol consumption can decrease bone mass, and heavy alcohol use can also make you more apt to fall.

Take additional measures to help avoid a fall. Remove clutter that might cause you to trip, and be careful about using sedative medications and sleep aids that can make you unsteady on your feet.

Possibly take medicine. Your doctor may recommend an osteoporosis drug for treating osteopenia if all three of the following apply to you:
- You're age 50 or older.
- Your T-score is between –1 and –2.5 at the hip or spine.
- You have a 10-year FRAX-estimated risk of at least 20% for a major fracture or 3% for a hip fracture.

If you have osteoporosis (T-score –2.5 and below)

Once you've been diagnosed with osteoporosis, your doctor will likely start you on a medicine such as a bisphosphonate, SERM, monoclonal antibody, anabolic (bone-building) drug, or hormone (see "Protecting your bones: Medication," page 38). Osteoporosis drugs can help you maintain bone density and in some cases improve it. Your doctor will continually reassess your bone density to determine how well the medicine is working and how long you should stay on it.

Just because you start on medication, however, doesn't mean you should abandon lifestyle interventions. Although diet and exercise won't reverse bone loss once you've been diagnosed with osteoporosis, they can slow it. Continue with all of the lifestyle interventions listed above—get enough calcium and vitamin D, do regular weight-bearing and strengthening exercises (see the Special Section, "Strength training and balance exercises for bone health," page 34), avoid smoking and excess alcohol consumption, and reduce your fall risks.

If your bone density is normal

While the basics of protecting your bones—such as getting enough calcium and engaging in weight-bearing exercises—remain the same throughout your life, there are different factors to consider as you get older.

If you are a woman at menopause

If you are a woman in the early years of menopause, you are probably in the stage of your greatest bone loss. All of the lifestyle recommendations above apply, and you should do the following as well.

Assess your risk. If you have reason to believe you're at elevated risk for osteoporosis (see "Know your risk factors," page 10), talk to your clinician about having a bone density evaluation. If you have conditions or take medications that reduce bone mass (see "Medical conditions and medications that can lead to bone loss," page 7), ask your doctor what you can do to counteract these effects.

Check your calcium and vitamin D levels. Meeting the recommended intake for these nutrients is a good start. But in addition, it's wise to have blood tests for both. Calcium tests are often part of standard blood testing, but you may have to ask for a vitamin D test. The level should be at least 30 ng/ml.

Re-evaluate your exercise regimen. Exercise can not only potentially build bone but also increase strength, flexibility, and balance. Now is a good time to incorporate weights into your routine, if you haven't already been using them. Another Harvard Special Health Report, *Exercises for Bone Strength*, provides a full program of bone-strengthening exercises, including two strength workouts, a cardio program, jump training, a running program, and yoga. Note that these workouts are intended for people who are still in the normal range for bone density or who have low bone density that does not yet qualify as osteoporosis. People who already have osteoporosis should check with their physician as to an appropriate exercise program. For one possible program, see the Special Section, "Strength training and balance exercises for bone health," page 34.

Discuss preventive medications with your doctor. Many medications can help prevent osteoporosis (see "Protecting your bones: Medication," page 38). Your doctor can help you determine if you should take one and, if so, which may be best suited for you.

If you are 65 or older

At this point, bone loss has tapered off for women. But for men, bone loss may still be high. Regardless of your sex, you are still losing bone as you age. All of the previous suggestions for bone maintenance still apply. In addition, consider these options.

Increase your calcium intake and get plenty of vitamin D. The recommended intake of calcium is 1,200 milligrams (mg) for most people in this age range (see Table 1, page 22). Make sure that you accompany it with sufficient vitamin D. (For more detail on recommended amounts, see "Calcium and vitamin D," page 21.)

Keep up your exercise routine. In addition to strength training, work on balance exercises, such as tai chi, to lessen the likelihood of falling.

Consider medication. Some drugs are used for osteoporosis prevention and treatment, while others are for treatment only (see Table 6, page 40). You may want to talk to your doctor about whether you should take a preventive medication and, if so, which one. ▼

Protecting your bones: Nutrition

A nutritious diet is just as important in later life as it was when your mother urged you to "drink your milk" to strengthen your bones. Along with exercise, nutrition is a cornerstone of bone health—and general health, too.

Even if you've been lax about eating right in the past, it's never too late to start making healthful changes. Although foods that are rich in the bone-building nutrients calcium, vitamin D, and vitamin K won't reverse osteopenia or osteoporosis, they can help preserve the bone you have and keep you healthier over all. The ideal way to get these and other essential nutrients is through food, but if you're a little short, supplements may help you get the recommended amounts—particularly for vitamin D, which can be hard to get enough of in your diet.

Calcium and vitamin D

Calcium and vitamin D have long been recognized as essential to bone health, as well as other important functions in the body. Calcium provides the building material for strong bones. Vitamin D helps your intestines absorb calcium into the bloodstream, which delivers it to your bones, muscles, and other body tissues.

While it's clear that we need calcium and vitamin D to keep our bones healthy, whether we should increase our intake expressly for the purpose of preventing fractures is a little more controversial. Two 2015 studies in the journal *BMJ* found that adding calcium to the diet, whether through food or supplements, increases bone density by only a minimal amount, which is unlikely to translate into a noticeably reduced fracture risk. This is why, for people with existing osteoporosis, nutrition is only one part of a strategy that also includes medication to strengthen bones and prevent fractures.

In part because the benefits of calcium and vitamin

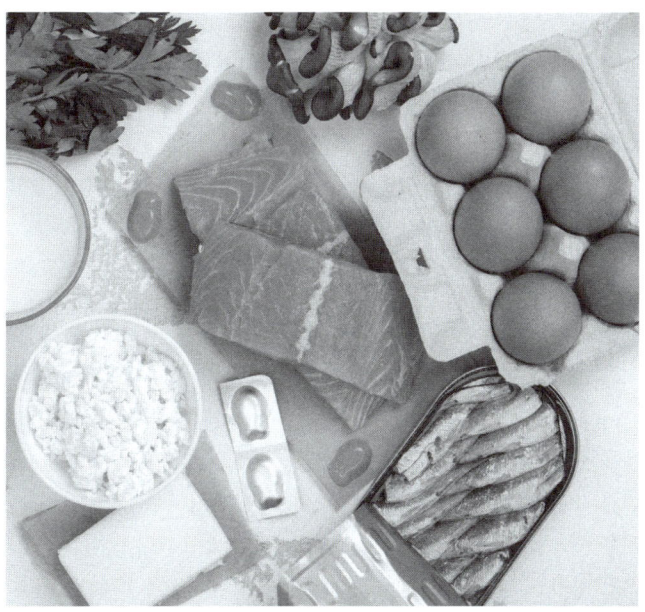

Abundant amounts of calcium are found in dairy products, but there is also calcium in salmon, sardines, and a variety of greens. Saltwater fish, eggs, and some mushrooms contain vitamin D.

D on bones and other aspects of health are still being worked out, experts disagree on how much of these nutrients we need at different stages of life. For this reason, in 2009 the U.S. and Canadian governments asked the Institute of Medicine (IOM; now called the Health and Medicine Division of the National Academies of Sciences, Engineering, and Medicine), a group of distinguished physicians and researchers, to review the evidence available and come to a consensus on basic daily requirements for these two vital nutrients. The 14-member IOM panel examined more than 1,000 studies and listened to testimony from various experts. The panel weighed the evidence for a range of health benefits—not just for bone health, but also for reproductive health, immune and mental function, and reduced risk of cancer, heart disease, and diabetes.

One key outcome of the review was a 2011 update to the Recommended Dietary Allowances (RDAs) for calcium and vitamin D, specifying the amounts that meet the basic health needs of 97% of all people at a given age. The RDAs for calcium and vitamin D appear in Table 1, below.

Controversy over the IOM recommendations

These recommendations were not met with universal approval, however. Some experts think that the IOM's recommendations underestimate the amount of vitamin D that people ages 51 and older should take to prevent bone loss and lower the chance of harmful fractures. The National Osteoporosis Foundation, for example, concurs with the IOM on calcium, but boosts the recommendation for vitamin D to 800–1,000 IU daily for men and women in this age group. Some vitamin D researchers recommend even higher levels. But the U.S. Preventive Services Task Force reviewed the existing studies and found no evidence that more than 400 IU of vitamin D a day was helpful for preventing fractures. The task force does not deny that higher levels could be beneficial—it only states that the current evidence is insufficient to prove it.

Why be so picky? Why not just take more than enough vitamin D, as a sort of insurance policy? One reason not to overconsume any vitamin or mineral supplement is that it requires time, effort, and money.

Table 1: Recommended daily calcium and vitamin D intake in adults

The Health and Medicine Division of the National Academies of Sciences, Engineering, and Medicine (formerly the Institute of Medicine) establishes Recommended Dietary Allowances (RDAs) for various nutrients, including calcium and vitamin D. However, its recommendations for vitamin D are lower than those of the National Osteoporosis Foundation, which are listed in Table 4, page 26.

SEX/AGE	CALCIUM	VITAMIN D
Women		
19 to 50	1,000 mg	600 IU
51 to 70	1,200 mg	600 IU
71 and older	1,200 mg	800 IU
Men		
19 to 50	1,000 mg	600 IU
51 to 70	1,000 mg	600 IU
71 and older	1,200 mg	800 IU

Source: Health and Medicine Division of the National Academies of Sciences, Engineering, and Medicine (formerly the Institute of Medicine).

▶ Calcium supplements: Harmful to the heart?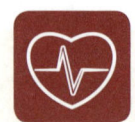

Some research has suggested that people who consume the highest levels of calcium from supplements may be more likely to have heart disease and heart attacks or to die from heart problems. However, any potential link between calcium supplements and heart disease remains controversial. People develop heart disease for a variety of reasons, and newer studies indicate that the connection to calcium supplements in earlier studies is likely to be a coincidence. A 2016 review of 31 studies, published in *Annals of Internal Medicine*, found no clear link between calcium intake, including calcium supplements, and heart disease risk.

National Osteoporosis Foundation guidelines say that up to 2,500 mg a day of calcium from food or supplements appears to be safe for the heart. And it's worth noting that *no* studies have found an increased risk among people who consume higher levels of calcium from food.

Ideally, you want to take what you need and no more. More important, taking too much of certain nutrients can be harmful (see "Calcium supplements: Harmful to the heart?" above). The IOM report set the safe upper limit for calcium intake at 2,000 mg daily. Excessive vitamin D could also be harmful, although you would need to take quite a large amount of it to get into the danger zone. According to the IOM report, the safe upper limit for vitamin D is 4,000 IU.

So what should you do? Here is a reasonable approach: Get as much calcium and vitamin D as you can from food (up to the recommended amounts), and make up any shortfall with a daily supplement. You can also get vitamin D from sun exposure without sunscreen, at least during the summer (see "Sources of vitamin D," page 26). If you are in your 50s or older, aim for 1,200 mg of calcium and 800 to 1,000 IU of vitamin D per day. And ask your doctor for advice if you are confused about mixed messages from the media.

Calcium in your diet

Most experts would agree that getting calcium from a balanced, nutritious diet is preferable to taking supplements. Foods typically don't have the side effects of calcium supplements, like constipation. Moreover, calcium-rich fruits, vegetables, nuts, and legumes contain many other healthy nutrients that can help protect you against heart disease.

Luckily, if you want to increase your dietary calcium intake, you have plenty of foods from which to choose. Table 2 (below) shows how much calcium is found in a number of common grocery items. You may be surprised at how much calcium you can add to your diet by making a few simple substitutions, such as choosing ricotta instead of cottage cheese, or opting for fortified orange juice over regular.

Many osteoporosis experts favor dairy products

Table 2: Calcium-containing foods

FOOD	CALCIUM (mg)	FOOD	CALCIUM (mg)
Cheeses (1 ounce, unless otherwise noted)		**Vegetables (1 cup, boiled, unless otherwise noted)**	
ricotta, part-skim (½ cup)	334	rhubarb (frozen, cooked)	348
Swiss	224	spinach	245
provolone	214	kale	94
mozzarella, part-skim	207	broccoli	62
cheddar	204	parsnips	58
mozzarella, regular	143	Brussels sprouts	56
feta	140	artichoke (1 medium)	54
cottage cheese, 1% fat (½ cup)	69	summer squash	49
Frozen desserts (½ cup)		cabbage	47
ice cream, light, vanilla	106	**Fruits and fruit juices (1 cup, fresh, unless otherwise noted)**	
ice cream, regular, vanilla	84	orange juice, calcium-fortified	300
Milk (1 cup)		blackberries	42
skim	306	orange juice, regular	27
1% fat	290	strawberries	27
2% fat	285	kiwi (1 medium)	26
whole	276	apricots, dried (10 halves)	19
Milk substitutes (1 cup)		raisins, dried (¼ cup)	18
almond milk, fortified	450	**Fish (3 ounces, unless otherwise noted)**	
rice milk, fortified	300	sardines, Atlantic, canned in oil, including bones	325
soy milk, fortified	300	salmon, pink, canned, including bones	181
Yogurt (8 ounces)		ocean perch, Atlantic	116
flavored, low-fat	345	trout, rainbow	73
plain, whole-milk	275	bass, freshwater	68
Nuts and seeds (1 ounce, unless otherwise noted)		halibut, Atlantic or Pacific	51
almonds, unblanched	70	anchovies, canned in oil, drained (5)	46
sesame paste, tahini (1 tablespoon)	64	**Shellfish (3 ounces)**	
hazelnuts	32	crab, blue	88
sunflower seeds	20	lobster, boiled	52
peanuts, oil-roasted	17	crab, Alaska king	50
Legume products (½ cup, unless otherwise noted)		shrimp	50
tofu, firm, made with calcium sulfate (¼ block)	163	*Adapted, with permission, from the U.S. Department of Agriculture, FoodData Central; Ohio State University Hospital, Nutrient Database Catalog.*	
soybeans, green, boiled	130		
navy beans	63		
baked beans, canned, with franks	62		

as a source of calcium. Dairy provides the most concentrated sources. Moreover, milk is often fortified with vitamin D. And the many reduced-fat milks, yogurts, and cheeses available today make it possible to cut fat and calories without skimping on calcium. In fact, these products often contain slightly more calcium than their high-fat counterparts do. There is, however, one potential concern about dairy that has not yet been resolved. Some research suggests that men who consume a large amount of dairy products may be at greater risk for prostate cancer. Because the men in these studies also ate fewer fruits and vegetables, it's difficult to tease out which factor—more milk or less produce—contributed to the risk. More research is needed to determine whether the bone benefits of dairy are worth the possible associated risks in certain men.

Many people avoid dairy for other reasons—most prominently, lactose intolerance. If you're lactose intolerant and have trouble digesting dairy products, try taking the enzyme lactase—either as a pill or in liquid form—to help you enjoy these foods without worrying about unpleasant side effects. You can even find milk that is lactose-free (but still has the same amount of calcium as regular milk) and other dairy products that already have lactase added. Or switch to soy or almond milk, which also have calcium added.

Dairy products are not the only sources of calcium in the diet. The plant kingdom is also calcium-rich, with spinach, dried beans, and nuts among the best sources. Their calcium content can't always be accepted at face value, however. For example, the oxalic acid in spinach and rhubarb binds the calcium in these plants so that the calcium isn't readily absorbed. Insoluble fiber, such as that in wheat bran, also reduces calcium absorption. (Soluble fiber, such as the pectin in fruit, does not.) Unfortunately, there is no easy equation for determining how much of the calcium content of a fruit or vegetable is actually absorbed.

Fortified foods are another option. Just a cup of fortified orange juice supplies about 300 mg of calcium, and three-quarters of a cup of some fortified cereals, such as Whole Grain Total, offers 1,000 mg.

Food labels, while helpful, often require translating. The label information helps you determine how much calcium is in the preparation, not how much you need. Packaged foods list calcium content as a percentage of the FDA's Daily Value, which is 1,000 mg for adults. However, if you are a woman age 51 or older, the RDA is 1,200 mg of calcium a day—not 1,000—so the percentages on the label will not be accurate for you.

To determine how many milligrams of calcium per serving a product contains, multiply the percentage figure in the Nutrition Facts box by 10. For example, if a product's food label says that one serving provides 20% of your daily calcium requirement, that means it contains 200 mg of calcium. (This works for calcium because the Daily Value is 1,000 mg, but it will not work for other nutrients listed on the label.) Also know what constitutes a serving. It may be not be the same as the amount you normally eat.

Calcium supplements

While experts recommend getting your nutrients from foods instead of supplements, you may find that it just isn't practical or possible for you to get all the calcium you need from your diet. In that case, a supplement can shore up your calcium intake and your bones. In fact, one analysis of several studies of postmenopausal women found that the women who took calcium and vitamin D supplements for at least two years were 23% less likely to suffer a spinal fracture.

The dizzying array of calcium supplements on the market includes pills, chewable tablets, flavored chews, and liquids (see Table 3, page 25). When making a decision, it's wise to consider cost, convenience, and how well your body tolerates the supplement. Most calcium supplements also contain vitamin D_3.

The calcium in supplements is found in combination with another substance, usually carbonate or citrate. Some products—typically found at health food stores—contain other compounds, such as calcium phosphate, calcium lactate, or calcium gluconate.

Calcium carbonate. This tends to be the best value, because it contains the highest amount of elemental calcium—the actual amount of calcium in each supplement. The compound calcium carbonate contains 40% calcium by weight, while calcium citrate is 21% calcium. Because calcium carbonate requires stomach acid for absorption, it's best to take this product with food. Most people tolerate calcium carbonate well. However, some people complain of mild constipation or feeling bloated. Some well-known calcium carbonate products include Caltrate, Viactiv Calcium Chews, Os-Cal, and Tums.

Calcium citrate. These products are absorbed more easily than calcium carbonate. They can be taken on an empty stomach and are more readily absorbed by people who are taking an acid-reducing heartburn medication. But because calcium citrate is only 21% calcium, you may need to take more tablets to get your daily requirement. Calcium citrate products include Citracal and GNC Calcimate Plus 800.

In weighing your options, check the labels of products to see what the serving size is and what the "% Daily Value" for calcium is. Then multiply the percentage by 10 to find out how much elemental calcium the product contains. For example, if the label says a serving of the product contains 40% of the Daily Value, it has 400 mg of elemental calcium.

Reading the labels with an eye toward cost and convenience may help you sift through your options. Would you find it inconvenient to take several tablets a day? How many tablets or chews does the package contain, and what is your cost per serving? While products that yield a high amount of calcium may seem to be the best bet at first blush, they may not serve you best. Because your body has difficulty absorbing more than 500 mg to 600 mg of calcium at a time, more of the mineral may go to waste (see "Spread it out," page 26). So while you may think that you've met your daily requirements by taking that 1,000-mg calcium pill, you may actually be only halfway to your target.

Here are a few other things to keep in mind when choosing and taking a calcium supplement:

- Generally, calcium pills are better choices than multivitamins, which tend to have small amounts of elemental calcium.

Table 3: Common calcium supplements

PRODUCT	TYPE OF CALCIUM COMPOUND	AMOUNT OF ELEMENTAL (ACTUAL) CALCIUM	DOSE SIZE*	COST PER SERVING**
Caltrate 600 + D$_3$ Calcium Supplement	Calcium carbonate	600 mg	1 tablet	7–16 cents
Caltrate 600 + D$_3$ Plus Minerals Chewables	Calcium carbonate	600 mg	1 chewable tablet	9–17 cents
Citracal Calcium + D$_3$ Petites	Calcium citrate	400 mg	2 caplets	11–13 cents
Citracal Plus D$_3$ and Magnesium	Calcium citrate	500 mg	2 tablets	16–25 cents
GNC Calcimate Plus 800 with Magnesium and Vitamin D$_3$	Calcium citrate malate	800 mg	4 tablets	32–33 cents
GNC Calcium 1,000 with Magnesium and Vitamin D$_3$	Calcium carbonate	1,000 mg	3 tablets	24–25 cents
GNC Calcium Citrate 1,000	Calcium citrate	1,000 mg	4 tablets	29–31 cents
Os-Cal Calcium with Vitamin D$_3$	Calcium carbonate	500 mg	1 tablet	6–10 cents
Os-Cal Ultra 600 Plus Caplets	Calcium carbonate	600 mg	1 caplet	8–10 cents
Tums (regular strength)	Calcium carbonate	400 mg	2 chewable tablets	9–11 cents
Tums E-X Extra Strength Antacid/Calcium Supplement	Calcium carbonate	600 mg	2 chewable tablets	13–15 cents
Tums Ultra	Calcium carbonate	800 mg	2 chewable tablets	10–13 cents
Viactiv Calcium Chews Plus Vitamin D and K Supplement for Women	Calcium carbonate	500 mg	1 flavored chew	10–12 cents

*Number of pills you must take to get the amount of elemental calcium listed here.
**Based on a sampling of retailers and sizes. Prices may vary.

▶ **Spread it out**

Your body has a hard time absorbing large amounts of calcium all at once. So it's best to get your calcium in doses of 500 mg to 600 mg or less, a few times throughout the day. To get the most out of calcium-rich foods and supplements, don't take your supplement with a glass of milk. Instead, take your supplement a few hours after drinking your milk or calcium-fortified orange juice; that gives your body a chance to draw as much calcium from these sources as possible.

- The National Osteoporosis Foundation recommends avoiding calcium products made from unrefined oyster shell, bone meal, or dolomite that don't say "purified" or have the United States Pharmacopeia (USP) symbol on them, since these products have tended to contain higher levels of lead, a toxic metal.
- Also avoid coral calcium, a supplement made from Japanese coral. Coral calcium supplements have also been found to contain lead, along with mercury and cadmium (a metal that has been linked to cancer as well as kidney and lung diseases). And although manufacturers have asserted that the body absorbs more calcium from coral calcium than from other supplements, no evidence exists to back up this claim.
- Because calcium, iron, and zinc supplements interfere with each other, take them several hours apart.
- Similarly, delay consuming calcium (either from food or supplements) for two to four hours after taking tetracycline antibiotics, since calcium can decrease the drugs' effectiveness. People with hypothyroidism (underactive thyroid) should avoid calcium four hours before and after taking levothyroxine, because calcium can interfere with this drug's absorption. Ask your doctor or pharmacist whether a supplement will interact with any other prescription medications you're taking.
- Don't exceed the daily dose recommended by the manufacturer, since doing so increases the risk for side effects.
- Vitamin D helps your body absorb calcium, but it's not necessary to take them at the same time. However, if you aren't getting enough vitamin D from sunlight, your diet, or your multivitamin, you may want to choose a calcium supplement that contains the vitamin.

Sources of vitamin D

Vitamin D is called "the sunshine vitamin," and for good reason. Your skin cells use sunlight to produce a precursor chemical that the liver and kidneys then convert into active vitamin D. Some people make all the vitamin D they need by going outside for a few minutes a day with bare arms and legs. (Don't wear sunscreen during this short time, except on your face to avoid the photoaging effects of the sun.) Keep your exposure time short—just 10 minutes or so a day—to guard against skin cancer. And if you're out longer than that, do cover up or apply sunscreen.

However, it's unlikely that sunlight alone will generate adequate amounts of vitamin D for most Americans during much of the year. For example, if you live farther north than 40° latitude (the latitude of Denver, Indianapolis, and Philadelphia), the winter sunlight isn't strong enough to enable you to produce significant amounts of vitamin D. Sunscreen, glass, and clothing also interfere with this process, diminishing your ability to produce the vitamin. People with dark skin produce less vitamin D than those with fair skin. And no matter who you are, as you age, your skin can't produce vitamin D as readily, your intestines have more difficulty absorbing this vitamin from food or supplements, and your kidneys convert less vitamin D to the active form that your body uses.

For this reason, many vitamin D experts would recommend that you not only follow the National Osteoporosis Foundation's recommendations for

Table 4: Recommended daily vitamin D intake in adults

The National Osteoporosis Foundation recommends a daily intake of vitamin D that's higher than the RDA. (For the RDAs, see Table 1, page 22.)

SEX/AGE	VITAMIN D
Men and women under 50	400–800 IU
Men and women 50 and older	800–1,000 IU

Source: National Osteoporosis Foundation.

Table 5: Foods containing vitamin D

FOOD	SERVING	VITAMIN D (IU)
Sockeye salmon, cooked	3 ounces	447
Tuna fish, canned in water, drained	3 ounces	154
Orange juice, fortified	1 cup	137*
Whole milk, fortified	1 cup	124*
Almond, soy, or rice milk, fortified	1 cup	120*
Yogurt, fortified	6 ounces	80*
Sardines, canned in oil	2 sardines	46
Beef liver, cooked	3 ounces	42
Egg	1 large	41
Ready-to-eat breakfast cereal, fortified	1 cup (without milk)	40*

*Levels of vitamin D in fortified products may vary; check the label.
Sources: National Institutes of Health, Office of Dietary Supplements; U.S. Department of Agriculture, FoodData Central.

vitamin D intake (see Table 4, page 26), but also have your blood tested for vitamin D to gauge how much is actually getting into your system.

Vitamin D in your diet

You can try to make up for the shortfall with your diet, but only a few foods—such as eggs, saltwater fish, and liver—naturally contain vitamin D (see Table 5, above). Mushrooms have vitamin D if they've been exposed to sunlight, but don't assume they contain it unless the packaging says so.

In the United States, milk is fortified with this vitamin; an 8-ounce glass should have about 100 IU or more. In addition, the FDA has approved the use of a particular type of yeast that can quadruple vitamin D levels in bread. A slice of bread should have roughly 100 IU or more, if it's labeled "rich in" or "an excellent source of" vitamin D.

Vitamin D supplements

Given the difficulties of obtaining adequate vitamin D from the sun and food, most people find they need to supplement. Vitamin D_3, or cholecalciferol, is the form most easily absorbed and used by the body, so choose a product with D_3 if possible.

Most multivitamins contain 400, 1,000, or 2,000 IU of vitamin D, but 1,000 IU is the most popular dosage. Check the amount of vitamin D carefully. If it's low, you may need to add an additional source, such as a vitamin D capsule or a teaspoon of cod-liver oil. Just don't overdo it. A 2015 study sponsored by the National Institutes of Health found that women who took ultra-high-dose vitamin D supplements (50,000 IU daily for 15 days, followed by 50,000 IU every 15 days for a year) had no difference in bone density scores for the lumbar spine, total hip, femoral neck, or total body compared with women who took low-dose supplements or a dummy pill. Although their bodies absorbed more calcium, the increase was slight. It's not wise to double up on your multivitamins either, since that will deliver unhealthy amounts of other nutrients, such as vitamin A, which can actually lower bone density (see "Potential dietary dangers," page 28).

Vitamin K

You know that calcium and vitamin D are good for your bones, but did you know that the vitamin K in leafy greens may also help keep them strong? Vitamin K helps your body produce osteocalcin, a protein that is instrumental in bone formation. It also blocks substances that break down bone and helps regulate calcium excretion from the body in urine. Furthermore, research has shown that people deficient in vitamin K tend to have lower bone strength and are more prone to fractures.

For example, in a review of 13 studies in *Annals of Internal Medicine*, most of the studies showed that taking vitamin K increased bone density. Seven trials found a lower risk of fractures in Japanese people taking the form of vitamin K called menaquinone (vitamin K_2), a popular osteoporosis treatment in Japan.

That's not the only evidence. In the Nurses' Health Study, women who got at least 100 micrograms (mcg) of vitamin K a day were 30% less likely to break a hip than women who got less. Similarly, in the Framingham Heart Study, people who got the most vitamin K were less likely to break a hip than those who got the least.

Vitamin K in your diet

Current recommendations call for 120 mcg of vitamin K per day for men and 90 mcg for women. Most diets easily supply this amount. For example, a cup of fresh raw spinach will deliver more than enough to meet the daily requirement, and so will a generous portion of cooked broccoli or Brussels sprouts. Other good sources of vitamin K include collard greens and other green leafy vegetables. If you don't like those vegetables, try scallions, asparagus, or cabbage. Certain herbs, such as basil, sage, and thyme, also have significant amounts of vitamin K.

Some people have to be careful with vitamin K, however. If you take anticoagulants like warfarin (Coumadin), it's particularly important to keep your vitamin K intake consistent from day to day, since this vitamin influences blood clotting. If you take an anticoagulant, ask your doctor if you should avoid foods rich in vitamin K and supplements that contain it. (Note that vitamin K is in some calcium preparations.)

Potential dietary dangers

Researchers have identified some components of a typical American diet that may compromise bone health. In some cases, the science is not absolutely clear on how much of these foods is harmful. However, the evidence is strong enough that anyone who is at risk of low bone density—postmenopausal women, for example—might consider how much of these substances they take in. After all, it's easier to preserve bone than to rebuild it once it's lost.

Caffeine. Some preliminary research suggests that drinking four or more cups of coffee a day can put you at greater risk of breaking a bone. However, drinking two or three cups might reduce risk. It seems that taking in high levels of caffeine increases calcium excretion by the kidneys. More study is needed, but in the meantime you may want to forgo that fourth cup.

Salt. In addition to raising blood pressure, too much sodium in your diet can increase the amount of calcium your body excretes in urine. Following nutritional guidelines by consuming no more than 2,300 mg daily can help prevent this effect. So can eating foods high in potassium, such as bananas, avocados, and leafy green vegetables.

Protein. Some experts believe that high levels of protein, particularly protein from animal sources, may raise the acidity of the body, causing calcium to leach from your bones in order to neutralize the acidity. This issue is still being investigated, and there is no consensus on how much protein may be harmful to bones—if there is such a threshold at all.

Alcohol. Heavy drinking seems to sap calcium from bones and interfere with production of vitamin D (see "Excess alcohol consumption," page 11).

Soda. Soft drinks—with or without sugar in them—affect the body's calcium stores because the phosphate in soda interferes with the absorption of calcium from foods. If the soda is caffeinated, that compounds the trouble, as the caffeine increases the amount of calcium removed.

Vitamin A. Several studies have found a link between high vitamin A intake and fractures. Currently, the recommended daily amount of vitamin A is 700 mcg for women and 900 mcg for men. You can get vitamin A as preformed vitamin A or as its precursor, the nutrient beta carotene (which the body converts into vitamin A). Beta carotene has not been linked to fractures and is therefore a safer way to fulfill your vitamin A requirements. If you take a multivitamin, check to make sure that a significant part of its vitamin A comes from beta carotene. Also, avoid taking high-potency vitamin A supplements. ▼

Protecting your bones: Exercise

Exercise plays a dual role in fighting the effects of osteoporosis. First, it can help preserve the bone strength you still have. Second, it improves coordination and balance, which can prevent the falls that could lead to fractures. A study by Harvard researchers found that women who walked more than four hours per week had a significantly lower risk of hip fractures than women who walked less than an hour per week. While exercise, like diet, can't rebuild bone to the extent that medicine can, it might contribute to small increases in bone density.

However, bone health is not the only reason to work out. Regular exercise also lessens your chances of getting heart disease, lowers blood pressure, helps prevent diabetes, reduces the risks for colon cancer and breast cancer, improves mood, and adds years to your life. If these health benefits came in a pill, people would be clamoring for a prescription.

How weight-bearing exercise benefits bones

Weight-bearing exercise can significantly increase bone density during childhood and adolescence. The effects aren't as dramatic in adulthood. But it's helpful then, too, because movement that compels you to work against gravity stresses your bones enough that your body responds by reinforcing the bones that are under duress.

What exactly is weight-bearing exercise? It's not the same thing as classic strength training (also known as weight training or resistance training), where you challenge your muscles with weights or resistance bands, although some strength training exercises are also weight-bearing. Weight-bearing exercise refers to any exercise where your body is bearing your weight. That could include vigorous sports, such as tennis or running, which are options if you're trying to prevent osteoporosis. If you already have the condition, start with a gentler form of weight-bearing exercise, such as walking or tai chi. Talk with your doctor about the types of activity that are right for you. (Note that while swimming and bicycling are excellent ways to keep fit, they aren't weight-bearing, so they won't improve your bone mass or density but will help your muscles and endurance.)

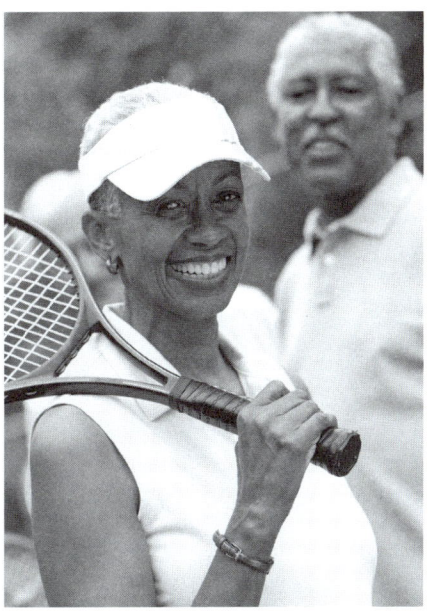

Any type of weight-bearing activity (in which you are supporting your body's weight) is good for bones, but high-impact activities like tennis give additional protection.

There are a couple of rules of thumb to be aware of if you're aiming for maximum effect on bone and you are able to work out vigorously. Generally, higher-impact activities have a more pronounced effect on bone than lower-impact exercises; sports such as tennis, volleyball, or running build bone faster than walking or low-impact aerobics. Velocity is also a factor; jogging or fast-paced aerobics will do more to strengthen bone than more leisurely movement.

Keep in mind that only those bones that bear the load of the exercise will benefit. For example, walking or running protects only the bones in your lower body, including the hip. That's why you also need a well-rounded strength training program that works out all the major muscle groups. This can benefit practically all of your bones, including the very sites most likely to sustain fractures from osteoporosis—bones of the hip, spine, and arms. (See the Special Section,

Beyond bones: Putting together a total fitness routine for overall health

Exercise delivers powerful, wide-ranging health benefits, but to reap its full rewards you must perform several different types of activities on a regular basis. Here are the various elements of a well-rounded program.

Aerobic. Each week, accumulate at least 150 minutes of moderate activity or 75 minutes of vigorous activity, or an equivalent mix of the two. Sustain activities for at least 10 minutes at a time.

Strength. Do strength exercises for all major muscle groups (legs, hips, back, chest, abdominals, shoulders, arms) at least twice weekly. Repeat each exercise eight to 12 times per set, aiming for two to three sets. Rest muscles for at least 48 hours between strength training sessions.

Balance. For older adults at risk for falls and others concerned about osteoporosis, include activities that enhance balance, such as tai chi or yoga, at least twice a week.

Flexibility. Do stretching or other flexibility exercises, preferably on days when you do aerobic or strength activities, or at least twice a week. Hold stretches for 10 to 30 seconds, repeating each stretch three to four times.

"Strength training and balance exercises for bone health," page 34, for workout ideas, particularly if you're new to strength training.)

To keep your bones healthy, aim to get at least 30 minutes of general weight-bearing exercise a day—reserving strength training with weights or resistance bands for just two to three days a week, with at least 48 hours between sessions. It's important to exercise regularly; infrequent activity won't strengthen your bones.

In addition to helping maintain bone density, exercise helps protect against fractures in other ways. Strength training increases muscle mass, which in turn enhances muscle control, strength, balance, and coordination. Good balance and coordination can mean the difference between falling—and suffering a fracture—and staying on your feet. Strong evidence shows that regular physical activity can reduce falls by nearly a third in older adults at higher risk of falling.

Classic strength training

Compared with other types of exercise, strength training can deliver the most benefits to the maximum number of bones. A strength training program typically employs equipment such as weight machines, free weights, and resistance bands or tubing. Not only does strength training protect against bone loss, but it also builds muscle and improves your body's ratio of lean muscle mass to fat. As a result, it deserves an important place in your exercise routine.

The Physical Activity Guidelines for Americans, issued by the U.S. Department of Health and Human Services, recommend strengthening exercises for all major muscle groups (legs, hips, back, chest, abdominals, shoulders, and arms) two or three times per week. Generally each exercise is done multiple times—for example, you might do eight biceps curls in a row. These are known as repetitions, or "reps." Groups of eight to 12 reps make up one set. Though performing one set is effective, doing two to three sets may be better. Give yourself a minute or more to rest between sets.

No matter what routine you use, the following tips for safe and effective strength training will help you get the most from your workouts.

Warm up and cool down for five to 10 minutes. Warming up brings nutrient-rich, oxygenated blood to your muscles while raising your heart rate and breathing. Cooling down slows breathing and heart rate to help prevent a sudden drop in blood pressure that can cause dizziness. End with stretches.

Focus on form, not weight. Align your body correctly and move smoothly through each exercise. Poor form can prompt injuries and delay gains. Many experts suggest starting with no weight, or very light weight, when learning a strength training routine. Concentrate on slow, smooth lifts and equally controlled descents while isolating a muscle group—that is, contracting and releasing the specific muscles that you want to strengthen.

Maintain a steady tempo. Tempo—for example, counting to three while lowering a dumbbell, then counting to three while raising it again—helps you stay in control. Too much speed and momentum can undercut strength gains and undermine form.

Breathe. Blood pressure rises if you hold your breath while performing strength exercises. Exhale as you lift, push, or pull a weight; inhale as you release.

Keep challenging your muscles. Begin with a weight that you can comfortably lift for eight to 12 repetitions. The right weight differs depending on the exercise. Choose a weight that tires the targeted muscle or muscles by the last two reps while still allowing you to maintain good form. If you can't do the last two reps, choose a lighter weight. When the complete set feels too easy, challenge your muscles again by adding weight (roughly 1 to 2 pounds for arms, 2 to 5 pounds for legs) or adding another set of reps to your workout (up to three sets). If you add weight, remember that you should be able to do all the reps with good form and the targeted muscles should feel tired by the last two reps. Most sporting goods stores sell dumbbells with adjustable weights, as well as wrist and ankle bands that fasten with Velcro and have pockets for weights. Look for sets that allow you to add weights in half- to 1-pound increments.

Practice regularly. Working all the major muscles of your body two or three times a week is ideal. You can choose to do one full-body strength workout two or three times a week, or you may opt to break your strength workout into upper- and lower-body components. In that case, be sure that you perform each of these components two or three times a week.

Give your muscles time off. Strenuous exercise like strength training causes tiny tears in muscle tissue. Muscles grow stronger as the tears knit up. Always allow at least 48 hours between sessions for muscles to recover. So, if you do a full-body strength workout on Monday, wait until at least Wednesday to repeat it. If you're doing a split strength session, however, you might do upper-body exercises on Monday, lower-body exercises on Tuesday, upper-body exercises on Wednesday, lower-body exercises on Thursday, etc.

Keep it up. As with other forms of exercise, consistency is the key to getting good results from strength training. As little as four to six months of regular weight training can help you maintain—or even improve—bone density. But people who stick with it for a year or more achieve the greatest gains. If you stop working out, any increases in bone and muscle strength will disappear within five years.

Safety first

A well-designed fitness program can improve your strength and mobility, but a poorly executed plan could actually lead to a fracture. With weak bones, it's imperative that you exercise safely. Here are some general guidelines to help anyone with osteopenia or osteoporosis make a smooth transition to a new workout routine:

Run the exercises by your doctor first to make sure they're safe for you to try. Getting your doctor's

Can yoga help prevent osteoporosis?

Could regularly performing a series of poses help preserve bone strength? A 2016 study in the journal *Topics in Geriatric Rehabilitation* suggests that a daily yoga practice might do just that. The study included 741 people, who were on average 68 years old when they started. Most had lower-than-normal bone density. After participating in a daily 12-minute yoga routine over a period of 10 years, the participants underwent DEXA scans, which revealed gains in bone density in their spines, hips, and thighbones.

While promising, the study applies to people with osteopenia, not osteoporosis. Many of the yoga poses used in this study involved spinal twists, side bends, and back extensions that help with prevention, because they place stress on the muscles around the spine. However, people who already have osteoporosis should avoid exercises that involve flexing the spine because they can further damage vertebrae that are already weakened by osteoporosis.

Yoga does have undeniable health benefits, including improved balance and coordination that could prevent falls. If you are interested in trying yoga, check with your doctor or a physical therapist first, to make sure it's appropriate for you and to be sure you know what poses are safe for your level of bone strength.

okay is especially important if you've fractured a bone in the past or if you have an additional condition, such as diabetes or heart disease.

If possible, book a few sessions with a physical therapist. Ask your doctor to write a referral for physical therapy. A therapist can go through each exercise with you, step by step, and check your form, so you can get the most benefit from each exercise with the least risk of injury. Keep going back to the therapist until you're completely comfortable doing the exercises on your own.

Pace yourself. No effective exercise program was created in a day. Start slowly, giving yourself time to adjust to the pace and movements. Gradually increase both the length and intensity of your workouts as you feel ready.

Avoid risky movements. Don't lift heavy weights. And stay away from any exercise that could end in a fall—for example, an unbalanced yoga pose.

Avoid spinal bends and twists. Be careful not to make any quick reaching or twisting motions, especially if you've broken a bone. You may need to modify certain exercises to make them safe or avoid them altogether. For example, to protect your vertebrae, forgo exercises and machines that put added stress on the spine, such as leg press machines, leg raises performed lying down, and squats done with weight bars resting on the shoulders. Golf swings and sit-ups also place stress on the spine and may result in vertebral fractures. Don't use your back as a fulcrum.

Don't overdo it. Expect to be sore during your early exercise sessions, but if you're in pain, ease back. You might be moving too quickly or pushing yourself too hard.

Tai chi improves balance, muscle strength, and flexibility

Evidence is growing that tai chi, a mind-body practice that originated in China as a martial art, has value in treating or preventing many health problems. Tai chi helps improve balance, and there is preliminary evidence that it may help maintain bone strength, too.

In this low-impact exercise program, you move slowly, without pausing, through a series of positions. Throughout these gentle movements, the muscles are relaxed rather than tensed, the joints are not fully extended or bent, and connective tissues are not stretched. Because you are standing and you shift your body weight from leg to leg, you get the benefit of weight-bearing exercise, which may account for the potential bone-strengthening effect—though the impact is much lower and thus the effect on bone is less than with more vigorous exercise. On the other hand, tai chi is slow and gentle enough to be easily adapted for anyone, from the fittest individuals to people confined to wheelchairs or recovering from surgery. Especially important is that it is safe for people who are elderly, frail, and out of condition—individuals at particularly high risk for falls and broken bones.

Although the research on tai chi for bone strength has yielded mixed results, one study in Taiwan found that longtime practitioners of tai chi had greater bone density at the hip and spine compared with people who didn't do tai chi. Another study found that bone density actually increased by a small amount in the hip and spine in people who practiced tai chi for 10 months. By contrast, those who didn't practice tai chi saw declines in bone density over the same period. A third study found benefits equivalent to 12 months of resistance training. A 2017 review of 20 randomized controlled trials concluded that tai chi may reduce loss of bone density in the lumbar spine and femoral neck.

In addition to its effects on bones, tai chi improves muscle strength, flexibility, and balance—all of which help you stay fit and avoid falls and fractures. It can also slightly improve aerobic conditioning, if it is done at a fairly rapid pace and is challenging enough. What's more, tai chi doesn't require any special equipment or facilities. Here is more detail on tai chi's benefits:

Muscle strength. Even without the assistance of weights or resistance bands, tai chi can help build muscle strength in the lower and upper extremities as well as the core muscles of the back and abdomen.

Flexibility. Tai chi significantly boosts upper- and lower-body flexibility.

Balance. Not only does tai chi help keep you from losing your balance, but if you do stumble, the muscle strength and flexibility you gain from tai chi can help you recover before a stumble turns into a fall.

Proprioception. Proprioception is the ability to sense the position of one's body in space, and it declines with age. Tai chi helps train this sense, which is a function of sensory neurons in the inner ear and stretch receptors in the muscles and ligaments.

Aerobic conditioning. Depending on the speed and size of the movements, tai chi can provide some aerobic benefits. But to meet government fitness guidelines and get full cardiovascular and other health benefits, you're better off relying on standard aerobic activities, such as brisk walking.

Exercises and other measures to help prevent falls

In essence, the treatment and prevention of osteoporosis is aimed at a single goal: to forestall the fractures that can threaten independence, steal mobility, trigger depression, and result in pain, disability, or even death. You can do that either by fighting bone loss or by preventing the falls that often lead to fractures—or better yet, by doing both. Falling is one of the biggest causes of fractures, particularly among older people. More than 95% of hip fractures result from a spill. Therefore, researchers, doctors, and medical organizations focus quite a bit on this subject.

Two important ways of reducing falls are by improving your balance and enhancing your ability to react quickly to anything that threatens to upset your balance. Various types of exercise can help.

Balance exercises. All people are more susceptible to falls as they age, but women are even more likely than men to fall. You can help reduce the threat of falls by practicing exercises that improve your balance. (For specific examples, see "Balance exercises," page 37.) If you are already doing some strength training, you may find that many of your current exercises are helpful for improving balance as well, because they strengthen muscles that you use to maintain balance. Similarly, tai chi—which uses a long series of slow, flowing motions—can help improve your balance (see "Tai chi improves balance, muscle strength, and flexibility," page 32).

Power training. In addition to balance exercises, power exercises (strength exercises that emphasize speed) can help reduce falls by improving your reaction time if you start to trip or lose your balance. The strength exercises in the Special Section of this report (see page 34) all include variations that emphasize power.

10 more ways to prevent falls

Exercise is not the only thing you should do to prevent falls. Falls can result from a host of factors, some health-related and some environmental, such as failing vision or hearing, dizziness (sometimes caused by medications), bad lighting, wet floors, and obstacles in pathways. Here are some simple changes you can make around the house to minimize your risk of falling:

1. Clear your floors of clutter and any items that could trip you up, including loose wires, cords, and throw rugs.
2. Make sure that stairways, entrances, and walkways are well lit, and install night lights in your bedroom and bathroom.
3. Clean up spills immediately.
4. Wear rubber-soled shoes for better traction. Avoid walking around in socks.
5. Limit your intake of alcohol.
6. Keep items that you use often in easy-to-reach cabinets. Also, consider using reaching and grasping tools to get at difficult-to-reach items.
7. Add grab bars to your tub, and use nonskid mats on bathroom floors.
8. Be careful when pets are nearby. Tripping over a pet, most often a dog or cat, is a common cause of falls.
9. Talk to your doctor about whether any medications you are taking can cause dizziness or impair balance.
10. Have your eyes checked regularly.

Vibrating platforms: Do they help people who are unable to exercise?

A therapy called whole body vibration is being promoted as a way to prevent bone loss in people who are too frail or too incapacitated to exercise. The idea is that by standing on a vibrating platform, a person experiences barely perceptible vibrations that travel up through the soles of the feet. These vibrations cause muscle cells to react as they would to common activities such as standing, keeping balance, and walking. They twitch in sequence, making tiny contractions that exert small stresses on bones, resulting in increased bone density and muscle mass.

But the platforms can be expensive, and research on vibration therapy has produced inconsistent results. Some studies in postmenopausal women, with or without osteoporosis, have shown improvement or stabilization in bone density. Others have shown no effect. A 2015 review of studies on vibrating platforms for postmenopausal osteoporosis concluded that more research is needed to determine the mechanisms behind this therapy's potential effects on bone. And while the authors say a vibrating platform might provide some benefits when used as an add-on therapy, it is no substitute for standard treatments like bone-building medications and a bone-healthy diet.

SPECIAL SECTION

Strength training and balance exercises for bone health

"What type of exercise program should I follow?" This is one of the most common questions doctors hear from patients who have concerns about thinning bones. They are aware that exercise can play a role in slowing bone loss, but they don't know what type of exercise is best.

The short answer is any exercise that challenges your bones with weight or resistance. (See "Protecting your bones: Exercise," page 29, for more detail.) A well-rounded strength training program that works all the major muscle groups is most effective. This creates stresses on bones throughout the body, stimulating extra deposits of calcium and nudging bone-forming cells into action. The bones that benefit are those that attach to the muscles that are being worked. For example, the standing calf raise (page 35) benefits your shin bones. The bridge is good for the hips and spine. Finally, strength training—particularly if it includes work on power and balance—enhances stability, which can help protect you from falling.

Like most strength training routines, the workout presented here calls for doing each exercise eight to 12 times, or repetitions ("reps"). Those repetitions make up one set. Typically, in a complete workout, you will do two to four sets each of approximately eight to 12 exercises that, combined, exercise all the major muscle groups. This workout does that. Each of these exercises includes a "power move"—a variation designed to enhance speed as well as strength. In addition, at the end, we've included a few exercises that directly target balance.

Our workout is designed for older adults and people who are new to strength training. Still, it's wise to talk to your doctor before trying these exercises, particularly if you've been diagnosed with osteoporosis.

For the best results, do this workout two or three times a week, allowing at least 48 hours for your muscles to recover between workouts. For the greatest overall health benefits, also try to get 30 minutes of moderate aerobic exercise on most days of the week.

Note: This workout is adapted from another Harvard Special Health Report, *Strength and Power Training for Older Adults: Two complete workouts to start rebuilding your muscles,* by Elizabeth Pegg Frates, M.D. (Harvard Medical School, 2019).

Strength training and balance exercises for bone health | SPECIAL SECTION

Strength training exercises

All you'll need to begin this workout is a sturdy chair with armrests, a small pillow, athletic shoes with nonskid soles, an exercise mat, and appropriate weights. Begin by choosing weights that are as light as 2 pounds for your first few training sessions, so you can concentrate on good form. After that, add enough weight so the maximum number of repetitions you can do is eight to 12. If an exercise starts to feel easy, it's time to increase the weight you are using (within safe limits set by your doctor).

As you perform each of these exercises, remember to breathe out when you are lifting or pushing, since holding your breath will increase your blood pressure. As you release, breathe in. Rest for 30 to 60 seconds between sets.

For further tips on performing these types of exercises, see "Classic strength training," page 30, and "Safety first," page 31.

  Standing calf raise

Exercises the calf muscles

Stand with your feet flat on the floor. Hold on to the back of your chair for balance. Raise yourself up on the balls of your feet, as high as possible. Hold briefly, then lower yourself. Do eight to 12 repetitions. Rest and repeat the set.

▸ **Harder variation:** Once your balance and strength improve, do one-leg calf raises. Tuck one foot behind the other calf before rising on the ball of your foot; do sets for each leg. Or try doing calf raises without holding on to a chair.

▸ **Power move:** Rise up on the balls of your feet quickly. Hold briefly. Lower yourself at a normal pace. Do six to 10 repetitions.

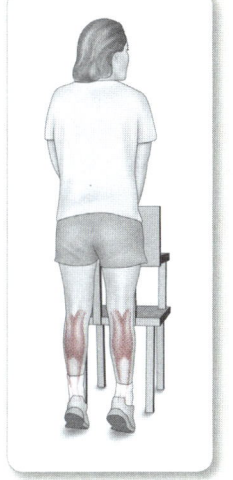

2 Stair climbing

Exercises the muscles of the buttocks and fronts of the thighs

Walk up and down a flight of at least 10 stairs at a pace that feels comfortable, holding on to the handrail for balance if necessary. Pause at the top only if you need to do so. Rest when you reach the bottom. Repeat four times.

▸ **Power move:** If your balance is good, go up the stairs as briskly as you can and come back down at your normal pace. Repeat twice for a total of three times.

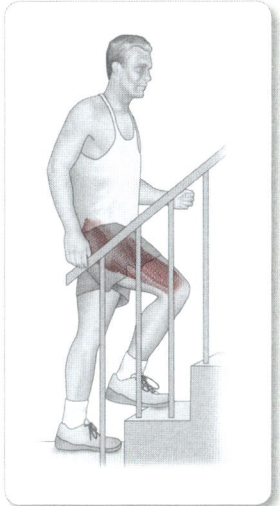

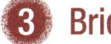 **Bridge**

Exercises the muscles of the back, backs of the thighs, and buttocks

Lie on your back on a mat with your knees bent and your feet flat on the floor. Put your hands next to your hips with the palms flat on the floor. Keep your back straight as you lift your buttocks as high as you can off the mat, using your hands for balance only. Pause. Lower your buttocks without touching the mat, then lift again. Do eight to 12 repetitions. Rest and repeat the set.

▸ **Power move:** Lift your buttocks quickly. Hold briefly. Lower your buttocks at a normal pace. Do six to 10 repetitions.

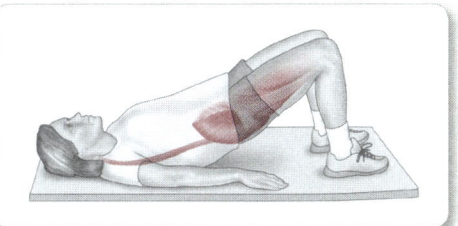

  Hip extension

Exercises the muscles of the buttocks and backs of the thighs

Wearing a weight on your right ankle, stand 12 inches behind a sturdy chair. Holding on to the back of the chair for balance, bend your trunk forward 45°. Slowly raise your right leg straight out behind you. Lift it as high as possible without bending your knee. Pause. Slowly lower the leg. Aim for eight to 12 repetitions. Repeat with your left leg. This is one complete set. Rest and repeat the set.

▸ **Easier variation:** Do this move without the ankle weight.

▸ **Power move:** Lift your leg quickly. Hold briefly. Lower your leg at a normal pace. Do six to 10 repetitions.

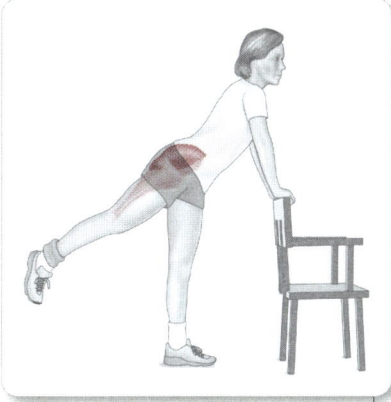

www.health.harvard.edu

SPECIAL SECTION | Strength training and balance exercises for bone health

5 Chair stand

Exercises the muscles of the abdomen, hips, fronts of the thighs, and buttocks

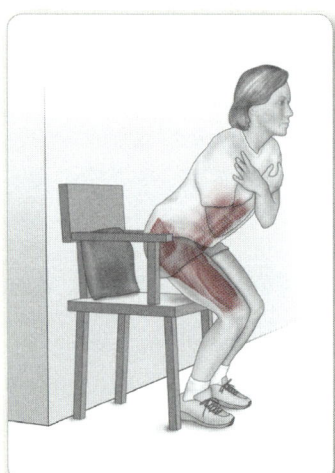

Place a small pillow at the back of your chair and position the chair so that the back of it is resting against a wall. Sit at the front of the chair, knees bent, feet flat on the floor and slightly apart. Lean back on the pillow in a half-reclining position with your arms crossed and your hands on your shoulders. While keeping your back and shoulders straight, raise your upper body forward until you are sitting upright. Stand up slowly, using your hands as little as possible. Slowly sit back down. Do eight to 12 repetitions. Rest and repeat the set.

▶ **Easier variation:** Use your hands to help you stand up.

▶ **Power move:** Rise from the chair quickly. Sit down again at a normal pace. Do six to 10 repetitions.

6 Triceps dip

Exercises the muscles of the chest, shoulders, and backs of the upper arms

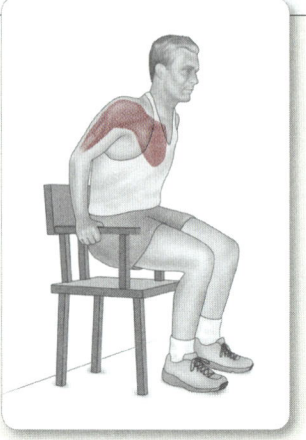

Put a chair with armrests up against a wall. Sit in the chair and put your feet together flat on the floor. Lean forward a bit while keeping your shoulders and back straight. Bend your elbows and place your hands on the armrests of the chair, so they are in line with your torso. Pressing downward on your hands, try to lift yourself up a few inches by straightening out your arms. Raise your upper body and thighs, but keep your feet in contact with the floor. Pause. Slowly release until you're sitting back down again. Do eight to 12 repetitions. Rest and repeat the set.

▶ **Variation:** If you don't have a chair with armrests, sit on the stairs. Put your palms down on the stair above the one you are seated on. Press downward on the heels of your hands, lifting your body a few inches as you straighten your arms. Pause. Slowly release your body until you are sitting back down again. Do eight to 12 repetitions. Rest and repeat the set.

▶ **Power move:** Lift your body quickly. Hold briefly. Lower yourself at a normal pace. Do six to 10 repetitions.

7 Overhead press

Exercises the muscles of the shoulders, upper back, and backs of the upper arms

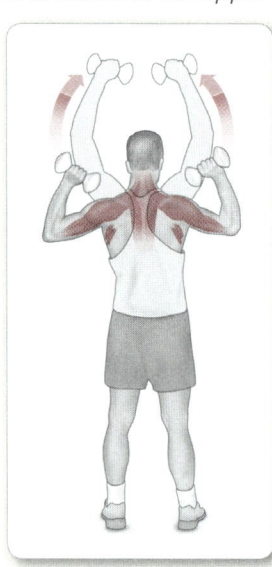

Stand with your feet slightly apart. Hold a dumbbell in each hand at shoulder height, with your elbows bent and the weights by your shoulders. Hold the weights so your palms are facing forward. Slowly press the weights straight up until your arms are fully extended. Pause. Slowly lower the dumbbells to shoulder level. Do eight to 12 repetitions. Rest and repeat the set.

▶ **Power move:** Lift the weights quickly. Hold briefly. Lower your arms at a normal pace. Do six to 10 repetitions.

8 Side leg raise

Exercises the muscles of the hips and sides of the thighs

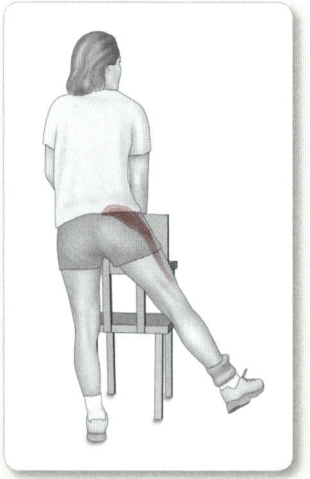

Wearing a weight on your right ankle, stand behind a sturdy chair with your feet together. Hold on to the back of the chair for balance. Slowly raise your right leg straight out to the side until your foot is about eight inches off the floor. Keep your knee straight and foot flexed. Pause. Slowly lower your foot to the floor. Do eight to 12 repetitions. Repeat with the left leg. This is one complete set. Rest and repeat the set.

▶ **Easier variation:** Do this move without the ankle weight.

▶ **Power move:** Lift your leg quickly. Hold briefly. Lower your leg at a normal pace. Do six to 10 repetitions.

Strength training and balance exercises for bone health | **SPECIAL SECTION**

9 Double biceps curl

Exercises the muscles at the fronts of the upper arms

Stand or sit holding dumbbells down at your sides with your palms facing inward. Slowly bend both elbows, lifting the weights toward your upper chest. Keep your elbows close to your sides. As you lift, rotate your palms so they face your shoulders. Pause. Slowly lower your arms to the starting position. Do eight to 12 repetitions. Rest and repeat the set.

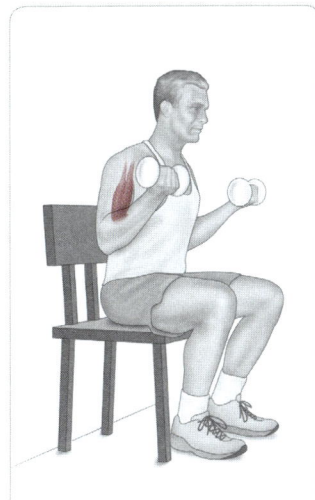

▶ **Power move:** Lift the weights quickly. Hold briefly. Lower the weights at a normal pace. Do six to 10 repetitions.

10 Reverse fly

Exercises the muscles of the shoulders and upper back

Sit in a chair holding weights about 12 inches in front of your chest. Your elbows should be up and slightly bent and your palms should be facing each other (as if your arms are wrapped around a large beach ball). Lean forward at a slight angle in the chair, bending from your hips and keeping your back straight. Now, pull the weights apart while trying to bring your shoulder blades as close together as possible. Let the movement pull your elbows back as far as possible. Pause. Return to the starting position. Do eight to 12 repetitions. Rest and repeat the set.

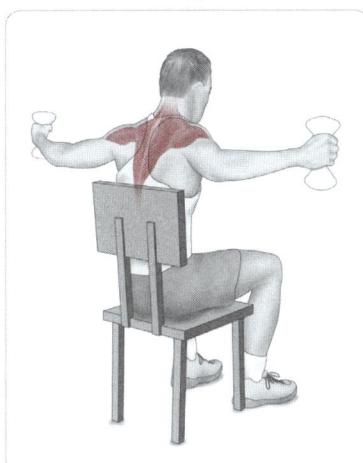

Balance exercises

An osteoporosis workout ideally has two goals—shoring up bones, and improving balance to prevent falls. Many of the previous exercises, including the standing calf raise, hip extension, chair stand, and side leg raise, are also useful for improving balance. But the following exercises are more specifically targeted at making you steadier on your feet.

1 Thigh raise

Wearing ankle weights, stand with your hands on your hips. Keeping your back straight, raise one knee up until your thigh is parallel to the floor (your foot will be lifted off the floor). Pause. Lower the leg to the starting position. Do eight to 12 repetitions. Repeat with the opposite leg. This is one complete set. Rest and repeat the set. Note: Ankle weights are optional, but if you use them for this exercise, they will provide added resistance and increased muscle strengthening.

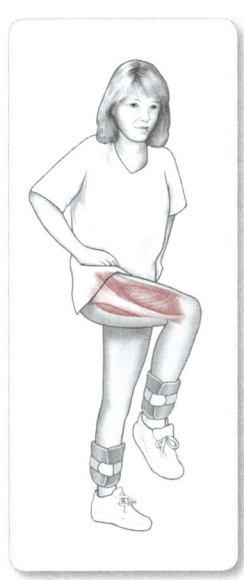

▶ **Easier variation:** Stand next to a chair and hold on to the back of it for balance, if necessary. Raise the knee that's farthest away from the chair up to hip height. Pause. Lower the leg. Do eight to 12 repetitions. Rest and repeat the set. Then turn your other side to the chair and repeat with your other leg.

▶ **Power move:** Lift your leg quickly. Hold briefly. Lower your leg at a normal pace. Do six to 10 repetitions.

2 Heel-to-toe walk (not shown)

Position your heel just in front of the toes of the opposite foot each time you take a step. Heel and toes should actually touch as you walk forward for eight to 12 steps. If necessary, steady yourself by putting one hand on a counter as you walk at first, and then work toward doing this without support. Repeat two to four times.

Protecting your bones: Medication

Nutrition and exercise can do some of the heavy lifting when it comes to maintaining bone strength, but medication also plays a key role, especially for women who have reached menopause.

Because medicines can have risks, they aren't recommended for everyone. According to National Osteoporosis Foundation guidelines, your doctor is most likely to put you on a bone-strengthening drug if you

- have fractured a hip or vertebra
- have a T-score of –2.5 or less at the lumbar spine, total hip, or femoral neck
- are 50 or older with a T-score between –1 and –2.5, and a 10-year hip fracture risk of 3% or more or a 10-year major osteoporosis-related fracture risk of 20% or more based on your FRAX score (see "How likely are you to break a bone? Your FRAX score and more," page 18).

This chapter describes the major types of medications used for osteoporosis. (A summary appears in Table 6, page 40.) Which one is right for you? That depends on your individual health status, fracture risk, and treatment preferences.

No matter which medicine your doctor prescribes, your goal isn't to stay on it indefinitely. The doctor will likely do repeat tests of bone density a year or two after you start the drug, and then every two years after that. You might also have blood or urine tests for biochemical markers that show how well the drug is working. These assessments will help your doctor determine whether and how much the medicine is helping, and if it's time to stop taking it or shift to another medication.

Bisphosphonates

Since the mid-1990s, when the FDA approved the first bisphosphonate, this class of drugs has become the first choice of doctors for treating or preventing osteoporosis.

The oral bisphosphonates typically used for

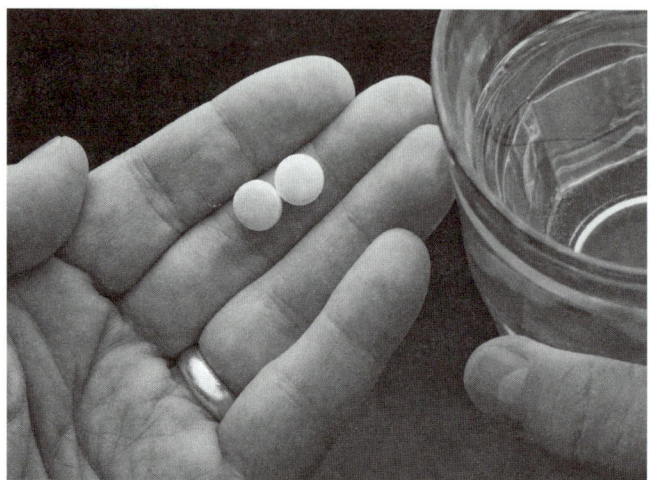

A variety of medications can help you protect your bones and even build greater bone density. Some of them travel preferentially to spots where bone turnover is high, such as the hips and spine.

osteoporosis are alendronate (Fosamax), ibandronate (Boniva), and risedronate (Actonel). Another drug in this class, zoledronic acid (Reclast), can be taken just once a year via an intravenous infusion that takes about 15 minutes. Like most of the medications approved for treating osteoporosis, bisphosphonates reduce bone resorption, slowing bone loss and producing modest increases in bone density. They accomplish this by binding to hydroxyapatite and interfering with bone-depleting osteoclasts. Osteoblasts then have an opportunity to fill in more of the trenches left by osteoclasts. As a result, bisphosphonates reduce hip, wrist, and spinal fractures. They became an attractive alternative to hormone therapy, which was once widely used for stemming bone loss but had fallen out of favor because of safety concerns (see "Hormones," page 46).

If taken correctly, oral bisphosphonates do not cause side effects in most people. But if they are not taken correctly, they may be hard to digest and can cause nausea, heartburn, or irritation of the stomach or esophagus (see "How to take Fosamax, Actonel, and Boniva properly," page 39). Many people find these instructions cumbersome. The inconvenience, coupled with the fact that osteoporosis doesn't have any symptoms, causes some people to question whether they need medication at all and to give up treatment. Others continue with therapy but fail to take their medicine properly. Experts hope that the development of more convenient formulations of bisphosphonates will help more people to take their medication as directed.

While bisphosphonates are usually well tolerated, some people taking these drugs develop severe or even incapacitating bone, joint, or muscle pain. According to a warning from the FDA, this pain can occur days, months, or even years after starting a bisphosphonate; for this reason, physicians sometimes attribute the pain to other medical conditions, resulting in prolonged discomfort and delayed treatment. While some people on bisphosphonates report that the pain disappears completely as soon as they stop taking the medications, others have found that the pain ebbs slowly or only partially.

Other reports have surfaced that bisphosphonates may be linked to unusual bone fractures, damage to the jawbone, or disturbances in heart rhythm. However, some of these effects remain unproven, and problems like these are very rare (see "How safe are bisphosphonates? A doctor weighs in," page 44). As with any prescription, you should report new or unusual symptoms to your doctor immediately. Let your physician decide whether or not the symptom is a concern instead of dismissing it yourself.

Alendronate (Fosamax)

Alendronate (which is available in both brand and generic formulations) is FDA-approved to prevent and treat osteoporosis in postmenopausal women, to treat glucocorticoid-induced osteoporosis, and to treat osteoporosis in men. It comes as a pill that's taken daily or as either a liquid or pill that's taken once a week. Another version combines alendronate and vitamin D.

Since 1995, when alendronate received its initial FDA approval, studies have consistently shown that it can slow or even halt bone loss, increase bone density, and reduce the risk for spinal and hip fractures. In a review of clinical trials involving a total of more than 12,000 women, treatment with alendronate reduced the overall risk for vertebral fractures by 45% and hip fractures by 40%, compared with not taking any medication. However, it's important to note that alendronate had this effect only in women who had already had a fracture before the study.

Alendronate is also effective for prevention. Studies have found that the drug increases bone mass in the spine and hip as effectively as hormone therapy, but without the same risks. It travels preferentially to spots where bone turnover is high, such as the hips and spine.

Studies suggest that alendronate is safe and effec-

How to take Fosamax, Actonel, and Boniva properly

Since alendronate (Fosamax), risedronate (Actonel), and ibandronate (Boniva) can be difficult to digest, people taking these medications orally must follow instructions carefully to avoid unpleasant side effects such as heartburn, nausea, or difficulty swallowing.

First thing in the morning, take the pill on an empty stomach with a large glass of water (at least 8 ounces) and then remain upright for at least 30 minutes (60 minutes for once-a-month Boniva). During this time, avoid eating, drinking, or taking another medication. It's important to take the pill with water, rather than coffee or orange juice, both of which can interfere with your body's ability to absorb and use the drug.

Most people tolerate these medications well when they take them as instructed. In fact, side effects are uncommon among people taking bisphosphonates in clinical studies, perhaps because study participants are more likely to take their medicine exactly as directed.

The consequences of not taking alendronate properly became evident a few months after the drug became available on the market. The manufacturer, Merck, notified physicians that women were experiencing more esophagitis, ulcers, and other gastrointestinal side effects than reported during clinical trials. The company attributed these side effects to patients failing to drink enough water with the pills or lying down in bed after taking them.

While bisphosphonates are quite effective in preventing fractures, the oral forms may not be the best choice for people who have recurrent heartburn, acid reflux, esophagitis, stomach ulcers, or difficulty swallowing. People who have Barrett's esophagus should not take oral bisphosphonates. If you have any of these conditions, ask your doctor about taking injectable or intravenous osteoporosis medications instead.

tive for at least 10 years. And it yields results quickly. A follow-up of the Fracture Intervention Trial, an important study conducted in the 1990s, found that alendronate was able to reduce the risk for spinal fractures within a year.

Furthermore, the benefits seem to linger even after people stop using the medication. In another follow-up to the Fracture Intervention Trial, researchers compared women who had taken alendronate for five years with women treated for 10 years. In those who took the drug for five years and then stopped, bone density showed a small decline but remained at or above where it was at the start of treatment. Moreover, fracture risk for the most part did not rise, except for

Table 6: Medications approved for osteoporosis

GENERIC NAME (BRAND NAME)	HOW IT'S TAKEN	APPROVED USES	BENEFITS	SIDE EFFECTS/COMMENTS
Bisphosphonates				
alendronate (Binosto, Fosamax, Fosamax Plus D)	Daily tablet or weekly liquid or tablet	Prevention and treatment of osteoporosis in postmenopausal women. Treatment of osteoporosis in men. Treatment of glucocorticoid-induced osteoporosis in men and women.	Increases bone density at the spine and hip. Reduces the risk for spine and hip fractures.	Difficult to digest. May cause nausea, heartburn, or irritation of the esophagus if not taken properly. Generally well tolerated.
ibandronate (Boniva)	Monthly tablet or quarterly intravenous injection	Oral version: Prevention and treatment of osteoporosis in postmenopausal women. Intravenous version: Treatment of osteoporosis in postmenopausal women.	Increases bone density. Reduces the risk for spine fractures.	The oral versions can be difficult to digest; may cause ulcers, nausea, heartburn, or irritation of the esophagus if not taken properly. The intravenous preparation may cause fever and flu-like symptoms.
risedronate (Actonel, Atelvia)	Daily, weekly, or monthly tablet	Prevention and treatment of osteoporosis in postmenopausal women. Treatment of osteoporosis in men. Treatment of glucocorticoid-induced osteoporosis in men and women.	Increases bone density at the spine and hip. Reduces the risk for fractures in the spine and elsewhere.	Difficult to digest. May cause nausea, heartburn, or irritation of the esophagus if not taken properly. Generally well tolerated.
zoledronic acid (Reclast)	15-minute infusion, given annually for treatment or every two years for prevention	Prevention and treatment of osteoporosis in postmenopausal women. Treatment of osteoporosis in men. Treatment of glucocorticoid-induced osteoporosis in men and women.	Increases bone density. Reduces the risk for spine and hip fractures.	May cause fever, flu-like symptoms, muscle and joint aches, and headache for several days after the infusion. Kidney function may be temporarily affected.
Monoclonal antibodies				
denosumab (Prolia)	Subcutaneous injection every six months	Treatment of osteoporosis in postmenopausal women and in men. Treatment of glucocorticoid-induced osteoporosis. Treatment to increase bone mass in women at high fracture risk who are takng aromatase inhibitors. Treatment to increase bone mass in men at high fracture risk who are receiving androgen deprivation therapy.	Increases bone density. Reduces the risk for spine and hip fractures.	An increase in infections, especially of the skin, has been reported. Transitioning to another antiresorptive drug after stopping denosumab may be desirable in order to prevent a rapid decrease in bone density and possible increase in vertebral fractures.
romosozumab (Evenity)	Two subcutaneous injections in a row, given monthly	Treatment of osteoporosis in postmenopausal women.	Increases production of new bone and bone density. Reduces the risk of spine and hip fractures.	Should not be taken by women who have had a heart attack or stroke in the past year. Because effects appear to wane and long-term safety data are lacking, should not be taken for more than one year.

a small increased risk of a vertebral fracture, and was generally comparable to that in women who continued to take alendronate for the full 10 years.

The researchers concluded that many women may be able to stop using alendronate after five years without putting themselves in greater jeopardy of breaking a bone. However, they noted that women at high risk of spinal fractures may benefit from continuing the treatment beyond that five-year time frame.

Risedronate (Actonel)

Like its cousin alendronate, risedronate is approved to prevent and treat osteoporosis in postmenopausal women, to prevent and treat glucocorticoid-related

Table 6 continued				
GENERIC NAME (BRAND NAME)	**HOW IT'S TAKEN**	**APPROVED USES**	**BENEFITS**	**SIDE EFFECTS/COMMENTS**
Selective estrogen receptor modulator (SERM)				
raloxifene (Evista)	Daily tablet	Prevention and treatment of osteoporosis in postmenopausal women.	Increases bone density, although not as much as the bisphosphonates. Reduces the risk for spine fractures. Reduces the risk for invasive breast cancer. Lowers LDL (bad) cholesterol.	Side effects are uncommon, but can include hot flashes, leg cramps, and blood clots.
Hormones				
abaloparatide (Tymlos)	Daily injection	Treatment of osteoporosis in postmenopausal women. Treatment of glucocorticoid-induced osteoporosis in men and women.	Increases the rate of bone formation. Reduces the risk for fractures in the spine and elsewhere.	Must be taken as an injection. Because effects appear to wane and long-term safety data are lacking, should not be taken for more than two years.
calcitonin (Fortical, Miacalcin)	Daily injection or nasal spray	Treatment of postmenopausal osteoporosis.	Increases bone density, but not as dramatically as any of the other approved medications. Reduces the risk for spine fractures.	Long-term safety is under evaluation. In the short term, the injected form can cause flushing of the face and hands, nausea, increased urination, and rash. The nasal spray can cause a runny nose.
estrogen (Activella, Climara, FemHRT, Ogen, Premarin, Premphase, Prempro, Vivelle-Dot, others)	Tablets and patches	Prevention of osteoporosis in women.	Increases bone density. Reduces the risk for fractures. Helps alleviate the symptoms of menopause, including hot flashes, vaginal dryness, and insomnia. Improves cholesterol levels.	Estrogen alone increases the risk for stroke and uterine cancer. Prempro, an estrogen-plus-progestin formula, increases the risk for heart attack, stroke, blood clots, and breast cancer; other estrogen-plus-progestin formulas have not been studied as extensively, so it is unclear if they carry the same risks.
teriparatide (Forteo)—synthetic parathyroid hormone, or PTH	Daily injection	Treatment of osteoporosis in men and postmenopausal women. Treatment of glucocorticoid-induced osteoporosis in men and women.	May double the rate of bone formation. Reduces the risk for fractures in the spine and elsewhere.	Must be taken as an injection. Because effects appear to wane and long-term safety data are lacking, should not be taken for more than two years.
Combination drug				
bazedoxefine and estrogen (Duavee)—SERM and hormone combination	Daily tablet	Prevention of osteoporosis in postmenopausal women and treatment of menopause symptoms.	Increases bone density in the spine and hip. Reduces hot flashes.	Side effects are uncommon, but can include muscle spasms, throat pain, and abdominal pain. The estrogen component of Duavee increases the risk for heart attack, stroke, blood clots, breast cancer, and uterine cancer.

osteoporosis in men and women, and to treat osteoporosis in men. It is available as a daily pill, a weekly pill, or a tablet taken once a month. Also like alendronate, risedronate has been shown to impede bone loss, increase bone density, and reduce the risk for fractures.

A handful of studies, including one randomized clinical trial, have directly compared alendronate and risedronate. In the clinical trial, once-weekly alendronate raised bone density in postmenopausal women more than did risedronate after a year of treatment, although both drugs reduced fracture risk the same amount. Like alendronate, risedronate works relatively quickly and helps to reduce bone loss and fractures in men as well as women.

Ibandronate (Boniva)

Ibandronate is approved to prevent and treat postmenopausal osteoporosis. It is available in a monthly tablet or as an injection every three months. Like the other bisphosphonates, ibandronate increases bone density and reduces the risk of fractures of the spine in women with postmenopausal osteoporosis. It has not been shown to prevent fractures in the hip or other sites except for the spine. Ibandronate has side effects similar to those of alendronate and risedronate, including heartburn, ulcers, irritation of the esophagus, and difficulty swallowing.

The quarterly intravenous injection of ibandronate is currently FDA-approved only for treating postmenopausal osteoporosis. Because the injected version bypasses the gastrointestinal tract, it doesn't cause the heartburn and esophageal problems seen with the oral bisphosphonates. However, the drug has been linked to short-lived flu-like symptoms in a small percentage of people.

Zoledronic acid (Reclast)

Zoledronic acid is a bisphosphonate given as a 15-minute infusion once a year to treat osteoporosis, or every other year to prevent bone loss. When zoledronic acid earned FDA approval in 2007, many women wondered whether they should switch to it. Not only was this new drug more convenient for patients, but it also showed an impressive ability to reduce fractures and boost bone density. In a study published in *The New England Journal of Medicine*, women with osteoporosis received either an annual infusion of zoledronic acid or a placebo. Over three years, the treatment reduced the risk of vertebral fractures by 70% and hip fractures by 41%. Women on the drug also tested higher for bone density at the hip and spine.

While these results are promising, some women taking zoledronic acid experience significant side effects, including fever, muscle and joint aches, and headaches for several days after the infusion. The drug may also temporarily affect kidney function.

SERMs

Bisphosphonates are not the only game in town. Bone loss can also be treated with a class of drugs known as selective estrogen receptor modulators (SERMs). These are often called "designer estrogens"—or estrogen agonists/antagonists—because they mimic some of estrogen's positive effects without also causing some of the negative consequences (see "Hormones," page 46).

In the body, SERMs attach to special proteins, called receptors, on the surfaces of cells, in the way a key would fit into a lock. When a natural estrogen molecule binds to such a receptor, it stimulates a response in the cell—and not always a good one. For example, estrogen can stimulate the growth of certain kinds of malignant tumors, including some breast, uterine, and ovarian cancers.

But SERMs don't fit the cell receptors quite as perfectly as natural estrogen molecules. That turns out to be good. It means that SERMs have different effects in different parts of the body, depending on the type of tissue—presumably because the estrogen receptors on these tissues are somewhat different. As a result, SERMs have positive effects on building bone, but without promoting cancer.

Raloxifene (Evista)

Raloxifene was the first SERM approved for preventing and treating osteoporosis. Unlike bazedoxifene (page 43), it is given as a single drug rather than a drug combination. Like estrogen, raloxifene slows bone loss; unlike estrogen, it does not increase the risk for uterine cancer, and it actually protects against breast cancer. Raloxifene is also approved to reduce the risk of invasive breast cancer in women who have postmenopausal osteoporosis or who are at high risk of breast cancer.

In clinical trials, raloxifene slowed bone loss and reduced spinal fractures by 30% to 50%. And in a major clinical trial, the Multiple Outcomes of Raloxifene Evaluation (MORE), raloxifene worked as well as tamoxifen (Nolvadex) in reducing the risk of breast cancer in high-risk women, and apparently with fewer side effects.

The MORE study also suggested that raloxifene might protect some women from heart problems. To explore this further, researchers launched the Raloxifene Use for the Heart (RUTH) study. The trial, involving about 10,000 women, did not find any change—either an increase or decrease—in the risk of heart attacks or other heart problems with the use of raloxifene. But it found reason for caution. While raloxifene did not increase the overall risk of stroke, women using the drug who did have a stroke were more likely to die from it. Also, the risk of blood clots in the legs was higher. On the plus side, the women were much less likely to develop invasive breast cancer or to suffer a vertebral fracture.

In its latest treatment guidelines, published in 2017, the American College of Physicians advises against using raloxifene for prevention of fractures. The report cites raloxifene's increase in the risk of blood clots and its failure to prevent fractures, other than in the spine, as reasons for this position. However, the Endocrine Society's 2019 guidelines disagree. This organization recommends raloxifene for reducing fracture risk in women with a low risk of blood clots who can't take bisphosphonates, and in those with a high risk of breast cancer.

One lesson from this research is that raloxifene, like estrogen, has wide-ranging effects on the body—some desirable, some not. If your doctor recommends this drug to you, make sure you fully understand the risks and benefits.

Bazedoxifene

Clinical trials of bazedoxifene, another SERM, show that it reduces bone loss and spinal fractures by percentages similar to those observed in studies of raloxifene. Potential risks are similar as well. Unlike raloxifene, however, bazedoxifene has not been shown to reduce the risk of breast cancer.

In Europe and Japan, bazedoxifene is available as a single-ingredient drug, but the only form approved in the United States is Duavee, a combination of bazedoxifene and estrogen. The FDA approved Duavee in 2013 to reduce symptoms of menopause, such as hot flashes, and to prevent, but not treat, osteoporosis in women who haven't had surgery to remove the uterus. This drug combination has not been shown to reduce the risk of fractures.

Women with a uterus who take estrogen alone for menopause symptoms face an increased risk of uterine cancer. Most often, such women take estrogen combined with a synthetic form of the hormone progesterone to offset this risk. The bazedoxifene in Duavee plays a similar role, discouraging excess cell growth in the uterus. Estrogen also can increase a woman's risk of heart disease, stroke, and blood clots (see "Estrogen products," page 46).

Monoclonal antibodies

Human antibodies, manufactured with genetically engineered cells, can block the activity of osteoclasts, the cells that break down bone. Two monoclonal antibodies have been approved to treat osteoporosis. They work in different ways.

Denosumab (Prolia)

The FDA approved denosumab in 2010 for treating osteoporosis in postmenopausal women who are at high risk of fracture. The agency later approved the drug for treating osteoporosis in men and for treating glucocorticoid-induced osteoporosis. Other approved uses include treatment to increase bone mass in women at high risk of fractures who are receiving aromatase inhibitor therapy for breast cancer and, similarly, for men at high risk of fractures who are receiving androgen deprivation therapy for nonmetastatic prostate cancer. It is not approved for prevention of osteoporosis. It is taken every six months as a sub-

Continued on page 46

How safe are bisphosphonates? A doctor weighs in

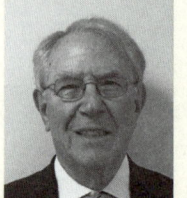

Media reports have fueled concerns about a connection between bisphosphonates and some troubling side effects, leading many women to ask their doctors whether they should continue taking these medications. To help sort facts from unfounded fears, Dr. David Slovik, medical editor of this report and an endocrinologist at Massachusetts General Hospital, answers some of the most common questions he hears from his patients.

Will Fosamax make my bones weaker?

Dr. Slovik: There have been reports that some women taking alendronate (Fosamax) and similar drugs experienced unusual bone fractures. This led researchers to question whether the drug may have weakened their bones. In these cases, it may be that the bisphosphonate decreases bone turnover (the process where there is some breakdown of bone followed by bone repair) to such a degree that the body is much slower in repairing microdamage that occurs naturally to bone.

Fractures may be related to dose and duration of treatment. The longer you take the medicine and the higher the dose, the more likely you are to experience an unusual fracture. Still, any possible connection between bisphosphonates and unusual bone fractures is unproven, and more studies continue to be needed. Even if the medications are responsible, that finding has to be balanced by the fact that these events are extremely rare.

Someday we may be able to determine who is more likely to suffer side effects from a particular drug. But in the meantime, it's important to keep in mind that more than two decades of research on alendronate and similar drugs has overwhelmingly concluded that bisphosphonates are highly effective at improving bone density and reducing fractures.

Can bisphosphonates damage my jawbone?

Dr. Slovik: There has been concern about a connection between bisphosphonates and the death of bone tissue (osteonecrosis) in the jaw. While no clear cause-and-effect relationship has been established, and scientists are unsure why some patients develop osteonecrosis of the jaw, there are good reasons to suspect bisphosphonates play a role. Just as with atypical fractures, the dose and duration of use play a role in osteonecrosis risk.

Most of these cases of osteonecrosis—about 94%—have involved cancer patients receiving intravenous drugs such as pamidronate (Aredia) and a type of zoledronic acid (Zometa) in doses much higher than are used for the treatment of osteoporosis. But this side effect also has been reported, with much lower frequency, in patients taking oral bisphosphonates such as alendronate, risedronate (Actonel), and ibandronate (Boniva) for osteoporosis.

It's important to remember, though, that compared with the millions of women taking bisphosphonates, the number of osteonecrosis cases is tiny. According to one estimate, the risk is between one in 10,000 and one in 100,000 per year. In other words, for every 10,000 people who take a bisphosphonate for a year, one may develop bone loss in the jaw.

Still, I think it's a good idea to have a dental exam and complete any necessary extractions or implants before you start taking a bisphosphonate. If you are already taking one, tell your dentist so she or he can consider it in planning your treatment. Also, be aware of the symptoms of osteonecrosis, which include pain, swelling, or infection of the gums or jaw; gums that aren't healing; loose teeth; and numbness in the jaw.

Is it true some osteoporosis drugs can cause atrial fibrillation?

Dr. Slovik: Atrial fibrillation is a common heart rhythm disturbance that affects more than two million people. Considering the millions of people who take bisphosphonates, it would be surprising if there weren't some overlap with this very common heart problem. Still, atrial fibrillation as an adverse event was noted in the initial zoledronic acid Pivotal Fracture Trial in 2007, but it has not been seen in other trials of zoledronic acid (Reclast) or other bisphosphonates. These initial results prompted the FDA to go back to data involving nearly 40,000 clinical trial participants who took one of these drugs or a placebo. Ultimately, officials didn't find a link between bisphosphonates and atrial fibrillation.

Meanwhile, regardless of whether or not you take a bisphosphonate, contact your doctor immediately if you experience any of the following symptoms: a racing heart, fluttering sensation in your chest, chest pain, or unexpected shortness of breath.

Do bisphosphonates put me at higher risk for breaking my thighbone?

Dr. Slovik: The controversy over whether bisphosphonate use is linked to thighbone (femoral) fractures dates back to around 2007 or 2008 when reports started to emerge of an association between these unusual breaks—in a location a little lower down than usual and occurring without the blunt-force trauma of an accident or fall—in women who had been taking alendronate for about five years. Since then, there have been other reports of so-called low-energy thighbone fractures in patients who had been on long-term bisphosphonate therapy. (Low-energy fractures occur from a fall from standing height or less.) Sometimes patients complain of achiness or pain in their thighs or hips before the fracture occurs.

Some researchers speculate that continued suppression of bone remodeling by alendronate and other bisphosphonates may have encouraged microdamage to the bone. In the short term, slowing bone resorption increases bone density because new bone formation continues. But over time it may impair new bone formation and reduce the bone's ability to repair microscopic cracks from normal wear and tear. Ultimately bone may become more brittle and less resilient to wear and tear. But at this point, the incidence of atypical femoral (thighbone) fractures is very low, particularly in comparison with fractures of the hip, spine, and other areas, and a causal relationship has not been established.

Should I consider taking a "drug holiday" from bisphosphonates?

Dr. Slovik: This is a very popular question among patients. Limited research on the subject has made recommendations challenging. Yet based on the available evidence, experts have offered some guidance on whether a drug holiday is a wise choice for postmenopausal women with osteoporosis.

The first study to suggest that some women can eventually stop taking the drug, temporarily or permanently, was the Fracture Intervention Trial Long-term Extension (FLEX) study, in which women who had taken alendronate for at least five years were randomly assigned to continue the drug or switch to a placebo for five more years. Those who discontinued the drug showed a gradual decline in bone density, but at 10 years their bone density was still above baseline. They had a slight increase in the risk for clinical spine fractures, but the rate of hip fracture, a far more serious injury, was the same in the two groups.

The HORIZON extension, which investigated the long-term safety and effectiveness of zoledronic acid in postmenopausal women with osteoporosis, found that women who stuck with six yearly injections had fewer vertebral fractures than those who switched to a placebo after three years.

After taking into consideration the combined results of these and other studies, a task force of the American Society for Bone and Mineral Research in 2016 recommended that doctors re-evaluate their patients after five years on oral bisphosphonates, or three years on intravenous bisphosphonates. For some women—including those who have a high fracture risk score, a low hip T-score, or a past fracture—it may be worth staying on the drug for longer (up to 10 years for oral bisphosphonates, and six years for intravenous bisphosphonates). Women who aren't at such high risk may be able to take a two- or three-year holiday after three to five years of treatment, without suffering significant bone degeneration.

Whatever you do, don't simply stop taking the drug without first talking to your doctor. Although we know that bisphosphonates stay in bone for years, we have little solid evidence to guide us in this area, so it's not clear whether a drug holiday will lower the risk for long-term effects. If you do decide to stop the medication, be sure to have your bone density tested after a year or two. If it has declined significantly, you can always resume therapy, although when to do so is unclear and awaits further study.

Can I safely take bisphosphonates after fracture surgery?

Dr. Slovik: Bisphosphonates are known for their ability to strengthen bones and reduce the risk of fractures. Yet there has been some debate over whether it's wise to take them shortly after you have surgery to repair a fractured bone. In years past, experts raised concerns that these drugs might interfere with bone remodeling and delay recovery. A 2015 review and meta-analysis of studies counters these concerns. The authors found that taking bisphosphonates had no adverse effect on fracture healing. And, they said the ability of these drugs to reduce bone resorption should lower the rate of fractures following surgery.

What's your overall take on bisphosphonates?

Dr. Slovik: Millions of women and men have benefited from bisphosphonates since they first came on the market in 1995 for the treatment of osteoporosis. Research shows that there's been a decrease in hip fractures. That is likely due in large part to the use of bisphosphonates, along with our ability to diagnose and treat osteoporosis earlier and with increased patient education. It's clear to me that these medications play an important role in building bone strength and preventing fractures. And in my experience they are usually quite safe. Major side effects are rare if they are taken properly, for the shortest time necessary to achieve the beneficial effect and with collaboration between the patient and physician.

Continued from page 43

cutaneous (under the skin) injection, like a flu shot.

Denosumab is a human monoclonal antibody that acts to reduce the formation and action of osteoclasts. It falls into a class of drugs known as RANK ligand inhibitors, but it is the only one used to treat osteoporosis. In clinical trials, denosumab reduced bone resorption, increased bone density, and reduced fractures in both men and women. It represents another option for people who have trouble taking oral bisphosphonates or other standard drugs.

Multiple spinal fractures have been reported in some people in the months after they stopped taking denosumab. This can occur because bone resorption may rapidly and temporarily increase (and therefore bone density may decrease) after the drug is halted. In 2017, the FDA added a warning on the label about this risk. It says doctors should consider prescribing another antiresorptive drug to reduce the risk of spinal fractures in patients who stop denosumab.

Romosozumab (Evenity)

Romosozumab, the newest osteoporosis drug, was approved by the FDA in 2019 for treating osteoporosis in women who are at high risk of fracture or who can't take other drugs for this purpose.

Unlike denosumab and most other osteoporosis drugs, romosozumab works by encouraging production of new bone. Romosozumab is classified as a sclerostin inhibitor, meaning that it binds to and blocks the effects of sclerostin, a protein that relays messages telling osteoblasts when it's time to slow down production of new bone. By blocking this chemical conversation, romosozumab tricks the body into producing more bone.

Romosozumab is given once a month by injection—two shots, one after the other. Treatment should continue no more than 12 months, because its bone-building effect wanes over time. After a year, a person can switch to another drug, such as one of the bisphosphonates or denosumab, to maintain bone density.

A two-year randomized controlled trial of this drug enrolled 4,093 postmenopausal women. Half of them received romosozumab for 12 months, followed by alendronate for another 12 months. The other group took alendronate for the whole 24 months. When results were tallied at the end of two years, there were 127 new spinal fractures in the romosozumab group compared with 243 in the alendronate-only group—and a total of 41 hip fractures in the romosozumab group versus 66 for women taking alendronate only. Women in the romosozumab group also gained more bone density.

Both drugs had similar side effects. The most common ones included joint pains and headaches. But the romosozumab group had higher rates of heart attacks, strokes, and deaths related to those events. This drug's label contains an FDA warning that it should not be taken by women who have had a heart attack or stroke in the past year, and that doctors should consider whether the benefits outweigh the risks in patients who have risk factors for heart attacks or strokes.

Hormones

Naturally occurring hormones can have important effects on bone. So can synthetic ones.

Estrogen products (Premarin, Estrace, others)

Many women use hormones in the years leading up to and following menopause to ease hot flashes, insomnia, and vaginal dryness. At one time hormone therapy was also widely prescribed to reduce menopausal bone loss. Its use for this purpose has fallen sharply, however, since the Women's Health Initiative—the only large, long-term randomized controlled trial of hormone therapy—was halted in 2002, after women taking a combination of estrogen and progestin were found to be at higher risk of breast cancer, heart disease, stroke, and blood clots in the veins and lungs.

Critics of this study say the risks were exaggerated. They point out that only one hormone preparation was used in each arm of the trial and that other formulas may not carry the same risks or benefits. Others note that the women who suffered the most health problems in the study began taking the hormones in their 60s and 70s, long after the start of menopause.

Nevertheless, the North American Menopause Society and other authorities advise caution, recommending that women limit their use of hormones to the smallest effective dose for the shortest period of time—and only if they have no contraindications (reasons not to take it), such as a history of breast cancer. Since by definition, taking hormones to preserve bone involves long-term use of the therapy, most doctors no longer prescribe hormone therapy just for preventing osteoporosis—especially since other drugs can effectively prevent and treat the problem.

That said, if you do choose hormone therapy to combat menopausal symptoms, you can expect a boost to bone health, since hormone therapy both increases bone strength and reduces the risk of fracture in the spine and hip—at least during the time you're using it. Unfortunately, as soon as you stop taking hormones, the bone benefit begins to fade, with bone density dropping back to baseline within a year or two.

Teriparatide (Forteo)

The FDA has approved teriparatide, a synthetic version of parathyroid hormone, for the treatment—but not prevention—of osteoporosis in both men and postmenopausal women and for treating glucocorticoid-induced osteoporosis.

Parathyroid hormone is produced naturally in the body and works in several ways to increase the amount of calcium in circulation. It promotes calcium absorption in the intestines and slows its excretion by the kidneys. While too much of the hormone accelerates bone loss, low doses taken intermittently can increase bone mass and strengthen bone (see Figure 9, below left).

Unlike medications that slow the rate of bone loss, teriparatide actually helps build new bone by increasing the activity and number of bone-building osteoblasts. And it can increase bone mass dramatically. One study found that teriparatide was more effective than alendronate in increasing bone density and decreasing fractures in postmenopausal women with osteoporosis. Teriparatide appears to reduce vertebral fractures by 65% to 70% and to reduce fractures at other sites by about 50%.

Because teriparatide builds bone while bisphosphonates reduce bone resorption, doctors have wondered if taking both drugs—at the same time or sequentially—would have a greater effect than either alone. Clinical trials on the subject are ongoing.

Teriparatide is recommended for people who have osteoporosis and are at high risk for a fracture. This includes people who have already suffered a nontraumatic fracture of the spine, hip, or another major bone. (A nontraumatic fracture is one that's caused by a fall from a standing height as opposed to an automobile accident or a fall from a ladder, porch, chair, or some other height.) This drug is also prescribed for people with multiple risk factors for fractures (such as a family history of osteoporosis, poor calcium intake, and a T-score of less than −2.5).

The drug is available only as a once-a-day injection, and it is recommended that treatment be limited to no more than two years. The Endocrine Society recommends switching after two years to a bisphosphonate or other antiresorptive agent to preserve or augment any gains in bone density.

Side effects can include nausea, dizziness, and leg cramps. Studies in rats have found an increased risk of bone cancer, but only with much higher doses than are used in people. Teriparatide has been around for almost two decades, and to date, no studies have shown that it increases bone cancer risk in humans.

Figure 9: Parathyroid hormone and bone

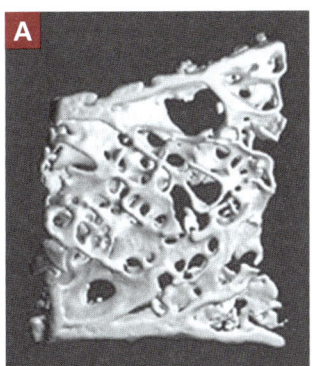
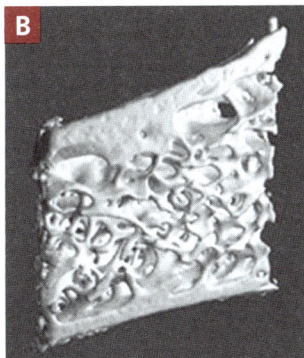

These pictures from a scanning electron microscope show bone biopsies taken from a 64-year-old woman, before (**A**) and after (**B**) parathyroid hormone treatment. Improvements can be seen in interior structure (microarchitecture) and outer (cortical) thickness.

Reproduced from Dempster DW, et al. Journal of Bone and Mineral Research (Oct. 2001), Vol. 16, No. 10, pp. 1846–53, with permission of the American Society for Bone and Mineral Research.

Abaloparatide (Tymlos)

Approved by the FDA in 2017, abaloparatide is a synthetic version of human parathyroid hormone–related protein (hPTHrP) that works in a way similar to teriparatide. Results show that this drug increases bone density scores for the lumbar spine, total hip, and femoral neck and that it also reduces fracture risk. One 2019 study suggests that both abaloparatide and teriparatide also improve bone quality, as measured by the trabecular bone score (see "Tests of bone quality," page 17).

Like teriparatide, abaloparatide is available by injection only. Side effects include dizziness, nausea, headache, palpitations, and excess calcium in the blood. As with teriparatide, abaloparatide increases the risk of bone cancer in rats, but there's no evidence of a similar risk in humans.

Use of abaloparatide should be limited to two years, potentially followed by an antiresorptive drug. In addition, the package insert suggests that the total use of teriparatide and abaloparatide (either or both) be limited to two years.

Calcitonin (Fortical, Miacalcin)

Calcitonin is approved only for the treatment, not the prevention, of osteoporosis. This hormone is produced by the thyroid gland, but its physiologic role in humans is not established. Salmon is the most common source of calcitonin used in medications. Taken as either an injection or a nasal spray, it inhibits bone resorption by osteoclasts.

Although calcitonin has been tested in a large number of clinical trials and has been used to treat women with bone loss for many years, it doesn't build bone as robustly as other medications. Women who take it usually see a slowing of bone loss or just a slight increase in bone mass. It reduces the risk for spinal fractures but hasn't been shown to lessen the risk for other kinds of fractures. There also is some evidence that calcitonin has painkilling properties.

People who take calcitonin by injection generally experience more side effects than do those who use the nasal spray version. Side effects include flushing in the face and hands, dizziness, nausea, rash, and increased urination. The spray formulation can cause nasal symptoms, including a runny nose or nasal crusts and irritation.

In addition to these minor side effects, a few studies found slightly higher cancer risks in people taking the drug. The data were not specific enough to single out particular types of cancer. But in 2012, the European Medicines Agency recommended that calcitonin not be used to treat osteoporosis because of the overall increase in risk. Canada's health agency took calcitonin nasal spray off the market in 2013. After reviewing the drug's safety, however, the FDA found insufficient evidence to justify pulling calcitonin from the U.S. market. Instead, it recommends that calcitonin be used only in cases where people can't tolerate or don't want to take other osteoporosis drugs.

If you're considering this treatment, weigh its potential side effects carefully when deciding.

Coping with fractures

Breaking a bone is often painful and frightening. Recovery can take months, and a break can threaten your ability to perform simple everyday tasks such as carrying groceries, making your own meals, or cleaning. But there is a lot you can do to recover from a fracture and prevent future breaks. The first step may be as simple as reaching out for help. Physical therapists, occupational therapists, and support groups can assist you. In addition, this section offers more information on how to mend your bones.

Meanwhile, getting enough calcium and vitamin D, performing weight-bearing and strengthening exercises regularly, taking steps to prevent falls, and using an osteoporosis medication can help guard your bones against future fractures.

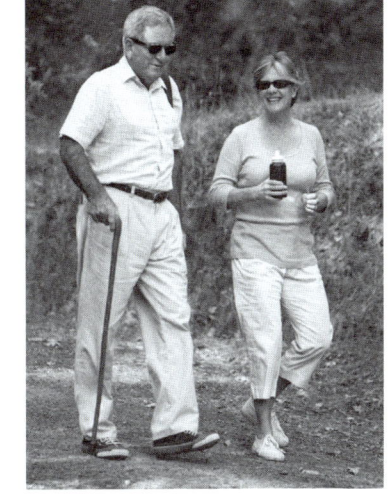

If you need a cane, hold it in the hand opposite the side that needs support, about four inches out to the side.

Living with vertebral fractures

Spinal fractures, which often take two to four months to heal, can be very painful. The most common way to treat pain is with over-the-counter medications such as aspirin, acetaminophen (Tylenol), ibuprofen (Advil, Motrin), or naproxen (Aleve, Naprosyn). Sometimes doctors prescribe stronger medications for pain, such as short-term narcotics. But be careful, as these medications may cause drowsiness, confusion, and a drop in blood pressure—all of which increase your chances of falling. Narcotics also may be addicting, even if taken for a short term.

Another staple of treatment is bed rest, although it should be short-term because prolonged inactivity can lead to further bone loss. Your doctor may also recommend that you use ice or heat packs to ease pain. Massage, acupuncture, biofeedback, and the use of a lumbar corset or back brace may also help for certain fractures.

If these interventions do not help (or don't help enough), there are two surgical procedures—vertebroplasty and kyphoplasty (see page 50)—that may reduce your pain, though both have potential side effects.

However you ultimately treat the pain, you will also probably find it useful to make some lifestyle adjustments. You may want to enlist your physical therapist's help in selecting a cane or walker, if you need one. He or she can assess your needs and help you choose the one that best suits your purpose (see "Easing the strain with a cane," page 51).

Exercise regularly, too. Talk with your orthopedist or the physician overseeing your care about what exercises are safe for you at each stage of recovery. Ultimately, your routine should include weight-bearing and strengthening exercises, which can build bone, and balance and flexibility exercises, which can make future falls less likely.

You may find that you also need to make a few practical changes around your house that will make it easier for you to maintain your self-sufficiency. An occupational therapist can give you expert advice. For example, if you can't reach the top shelves of cabinets any longer, he or she can suggest a number of solutions, from tools to help you grasp objects to ways of reorganizing your kitchen. An assistive device called a dressing stick can help people with limited mobility to put on and remove clothing without bending too much.

Finding clothing that fits correctly may also become a concern as your body changes. If you have had several vertebral fractures, you may notice that your ribcage has moved closer to your hip bones. As a result, many women find that their garments are too tight at the waist, while a larger size is too baggy in other places. Some women solve this problem by buying maternity clothes. The elastic panels in slacks and skirts are roomy in the front without giving too much in the back, and the loose-fitting tops are well suited for accommodating spinal changes.

Low-heeled, comfortable shoes that offer adequate support are also essential. There are many styles of walking shoes that fill the bill. If you have difficulty

Vertebroplasty and kyphoplasty

Two procedures are available to stabilize compressed vertebrae, alleviate the pain associated with this type of fracture, and improve daily functioning: vertebroplasty and kyphoplasty. These interventions are geared toward patients who haven't responded to traditional measures such as bed rest and pain medications. In addition, kyphoplasty may restore some of the height lost when a cracked vertebra gets compressed, or at least prevent it from getting worse.

Vertebroplasty is an outpatient procedure that takes less than an hour. After the patient is given mild sedation, the physician inserts a needle into the affected vertebra, using an x-ray as a guide. Then bone cement is injected into the compressed vertebra, filling the holes and crevices. The cement hardens in about 15 to 20 minutes, stabilizing the vertebra, creating a support that helps prevent any further collapse, and (ideally) alleviating pain.

Kyphoplasty (see Figure 10, below right) is a refinement of vertebroplasty. Like vertebroplasty, this procedure is aimed at stabilizing compressed vertebrae and relieving pain. Also like vertebroplasty, kyphoplasty takes less than an hour, although it may require an overnight hospital stay. In this procedure, the physician administers a mild sedative and then inserts a small tube-like instrument into the affected vertebra, using a special viewing device called a fluoroscope as a guide. Once the instrument is correctly placed, a balloon is inflated, creating a cavity in the bone. The balloon is then deflated, and the physician injects surgical cement into the void. The creation of this hollow minimizes the risk of the cement leaking and pushes the vertebral endplates apart, restoring some height.

Do these approaches work?

Reviews of studies suggest that both vertebroplasty and kyphoplasty reduce pain and improve function compared with lifestyle changes and pain medications. However, a lack of good comparative studies makes it hard to definitively determine which therapy is preferable. In addition, long-term comparisons of these procedures with standard treatments of bed rest, pain relievers, and physical therapy have not produced clear results.

Although uncommon, the potential complications of vertebroplasty and kyphoplasty include bleeding, infection, and nerve damage. Occasionally bone cement leaks from the treated area. If the cement enters the bloodstream or spinal canal, serious problems can occur. In addition, there is an increased fracture risk in the vertebrae adjacent to the one treated. The FDA has also warned that soft tissue damage, nerve root pain and compression, pulmonary embolism (a blood clot in the lung), and respiratory and heart failure have been reported among some patients undergoing vertebroplasty or kyphoplasty.

Given the uncertainties, it's important to find a physician who is experienced with the procedure and is willing to engage in a frank conversation about the benefits and risks. You may want to ask your doctor what type of cement will be used, whether it is currently FDA-approved for the procedure, and what experience your doctor has had with the product and the procedure in general.

Figure 10: Repairing a compressed vertebra with kyphoplasty

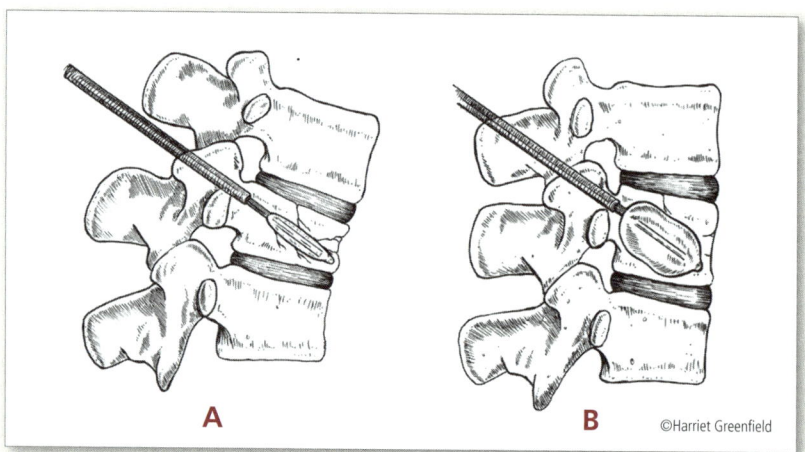

Kyphoplasty treats the pain associated with vertebral compressions. This technique restores some of the height of the treated vertebra. First, a tube is inserted into the vertebra (**A**). Then a balloon at the end is inflated and deflated, leaving a hollow in the bone (**B**). Finally, surgical cement is injected into the cavity, shoring up the vertebral endplates.

finding shoes that fit properly, you may want to have orthotic devices—supportive insoles that affect the distribution of weight—fitted by a podiatrist.

Living with a hip fracture

After a hip fracture, proper rehabilitation can make the difference between returning to active life and requiring long-term care. If the hip fracture doesn't heal properly, you may become limited in your ability to walk and function in an independent manner. Both physical and occupational therapy can be very helpful.

Physical therapists can teach you exercises to strengthen your hips, improve your coordination and balance, and increase your flexibility. A home visit with a physical therapist may help you transition from a hospital or rehab facility to a suitable at-home exercise program that can get you up and moving again and help condition your body to reduce the risk of falling. The therapist can also teach you safety measures that will lessen the likelihood of injuring yourself and improve your day-to-day functioning.

You should also schedule a home visit with an occupational therapist to eliminate potential hazards in your home—such as electrical cords and loose rugs in pathways, poor lighting, or a lack of handrails or grab bars. Also, talk to your doctor about other factors that can lead to falls, such as alcohol consumption or the use of certain medications.

Support groups

Osteoporosis doesn't affect only your bones. It can leave you feeling depressed, isolated, anxious, or afraid. You may worry about breaking a bone or losing your independence. Or perhaps you're overwhelmed by pain or upset by changes in your appearance. Maybe you are discouraged because you are no longer able to perform certain activities.

A support group may help you cope with these feelings and move ahead with your recovery. Talk to your doctor about finding a program, or check with your insurer, local hospital, or the National Osteoporosis Foundation (see "Resources," page 52).

Easing the strain with a cane

For something so low-tech and simple in design, a cane performs complex functions. You hold the cane in the hand opposite the side that needs support, about four inches to the side of your stronger leg. This redistributes weight to improve stability, helps reduce demand on muscles that may be weak, and takes the load off weight-bearing structures such as the hip, knee, and spine.

A cane can help you maintain mobility and ward off further disability if you have one or more fractures, as well as assist in recovery after surgery. So don't let self-consciousness stop you from using a cane if your doctor recommends that you try one.

A physical therapist or other clinician can help you select a cane, check that it's the proper height, and show you how to use it. He or she may also suggest certain muscle-strengthening exercises before you start walking with your cane.

Canes are available at medical supply stores and pharmacies, through specialty catalogs, and on the Internet. They generally come in standard, offset, and multiple-legged versions. Government or private insurance usually covers the cost of a basic cane if you have a written prescription from your doctor.

Standard canes. These are low-tech, lightweight, and generally inexpensive. They usually come with a curved or T-shaped handle and a rubber-capped tip at the bottom. Many people find that a T-shaped handle is more comfortable than a curved one. A standard model is good for people who need help with balance but don't need the cane to bear a lot of weight.

Offset canes. The upper shaft of an offset cane bends outward, and the handle grip is usually flat—often a

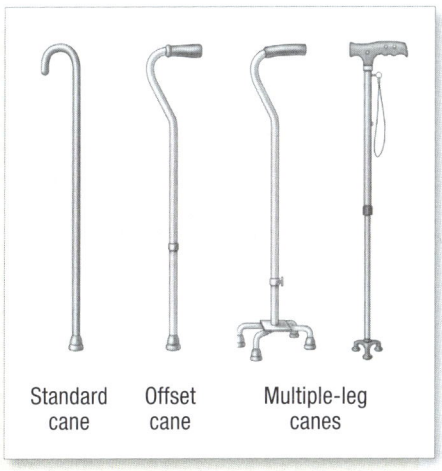

Standard cane   Offset cane   Multiple-leg canes

good choice for people whose hands are weak or who need a cane that bears more weight than the standard type.

Multiple-leg canes. Multiple legs offer considerable support and allow the cane to stand on its own when not in use. One drawback to using such a cane is that for maximum support, you must plant all the legs solidly on the ground. Doing so takes time and can slow the pace of walking.

Resources

Organizations

American Academy of Orthopaedic Surgeons
9400 W. Higgins Road
Rosemont, IL 60018
847-823-7186
https://orthoinfo.aaos.org

This medical association for orthopedic surgeons offers information on osteoporosis for laypeople. The website features fact sheets on such topics as keeping your bones healthy, recognizing the warning signs of osteoporosis, and preventing hip fractures.

National Center for Injury Prevention and Control
Centers for Disease Control and Prevention
1600 Clifton Road
Atlanta, GA 30329
800-232-4636 (toll-free)
TTY: 888-232-6348 (toll-free)
www.cdc.gov/injury

This arm of the Centers for Disease Control and Prevention focuses on reducing accidents and the resulting injuries and deaths. The division supports fall-prevention programs, and its website includes fall-prevention fact sheets and tips and an online fall-prevention tool kit for seniors.

National Institute on Aging
Building 31, Room 5C27
31 Center Drive, MSC 2292
Bethesda, MD 20892
800-222-2225 (toll-free)
TTY: 800-222-4225 (toll-free)
www.nia.nih.gov

This branch of the National Institutes of Health offers reliable, free information on osteoporosis for physicians and consumers. Publications are available on the website, or you can order them by mail or telephone.

National Osteoporosis Foundation
251 18th St. S., Suite 630
Arlington, VA 22202
800-231-4222 (toll-free)
www.nof.org

This nonprofit organization supports research on osteoporosis and develops educational programs and materials. Much of its material is also available in Spanish. Membership benefits include a quarterly newsletter, *The Osteoporosis Report*, which reviews the latest scientific information. You can order materials online, by mail, or by telephone.

Osteoporosis and Related Bone Diseases National Resource Center
National Institutes of Health
2 AMS Circle
Bethesda, MD 20892
800-624-2663 (toll-free)
TTY: 202-466-4315
www.bones.nih.gov

This information center is dedicated to increasing awareness of osteoporosis, Paget's disease of the bone, osteogenesis imperfecta, and hyperparathyroidism. The center was created to provide health professionals and the general public with information about these conditions and their treatment, as well as links to other resources. You'll find fact sheets, general information, and news about osteoporosis on the website, where you can also sign up to receive the center's electronic newsletter.

Publications from Harvard Medical School

The following publications from Harvard Medical School elaborate on topics in this report. To order, go to www.health.harvard.edu or call 877-649-9457 (toll-free).

Better Balance: Simple exercises to improve stability and prevent falls
Suzanne Salamon, M.D., and Brad Manor, Ph.D., Medical Editors, with Michele Stanten, Fitness Consultant
(Harvard Medical School, 2017)

If you have osteoporosis, it's important to avoid falls. This Harvard Special Health Report helps you learn how to do that by improving your balance and mobility, with safe, effective balance exercises that also increase flexibility, sharpen reflexes, increase muscle strength and speed, and firm up your core.

Exercises for Bone Strength: 7 workouts to help prevent osteoporosis and keep you standing tall
Elizabeth Pegg Frates, M.D., with Michele Stanten, Fitness Consultant
(Harvard Medical School, 2019)

If you do not yet have osteoporosis, but are afraid of developing it, this report can help, by offering a variety of workouts with proven bone-protecting effects—including two strength training workouts, three cardio workouts, jump training (plyometrics), and yoga.

An Introduction to Tai Chi: A gentle exercise program for mental and physical well-being
Peter M. Wayne, Ph.D., Medical Editor
(Harvard Medical School, 2017)

Mind-body forms of exercise, such as tai chi and yoga, have been gaining popularity. And studies show that they can help with everything from lowering blood pressure and managing depression to building strength and improving balance—a key skill that can help you prevent falls and broken bones. This report lays out the benefits and helps you create your own tai chi practice, including three simple routines for beginners.

Preventing Falls
Matthew Hamilton, M.D., Medical Editor
(Harvard Medical School, 2018)

Falls can lead to broken bones and even a loss of independence. But many falls can be avoided. This online-only guide from Harvard Medical School includes exercises to help strengthen your core and tips for removing hazards at home and learning to fall without injury.